New Developments in Medical Research

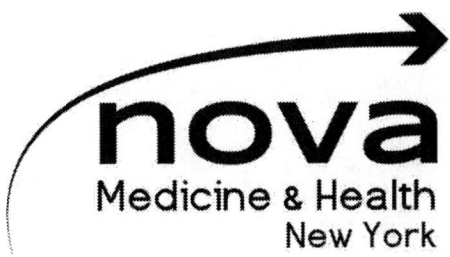

New Developments in Medical Research

Inflammation and Chronic Disorders: The Secret Connection
Ashwani K. Dhingra, PhD (Editor)
Priyanka Kriplani, PhD (Editor)
Bhawna Chopra, PhD (Editor)
Ajmer Singh Grewal, PhD (Editor)
Geeta Deswal, PhD (Editor)
Peeyush Kaushik, M. Pharm (Editor)
2023. ISBN: 979-8-88697-980-0 (eBook)

Antidiabetic Plants: Properties and Applications
Arpita Roy, PhD (Editor)
2023. ISBN: 979-8-88697-957-2 (Hardcover)
2023. ISBN: 979-8-88697-982-4 (eBook)

The Dangers of Psychoactive Substances
Denise J. Burton (Editor)
2023. ISBN: 979-8-88697-705-9 (Softcover)
2023. ISBN: 979-8-88697-712-7 (eBook)

An Innovative Program at Alfaisal Medicine: A Brief History and Guide to Success
Paul Ganguly, MBBS, MD, FACA (Editor)
2023. ISBN: 979-8-88697-638-0 (Softcover)
2023. ISBN: 979-8-88697-703-5 (eBook)

Botulinum Toxin: Therapeutic Uses, Procedures and Efficacy
James C. Lark (Editor)
2022. ISBN: 978-1-68507-817-1 (Hardcover)
2022. ISBN: 978-1-68507-826-3 (eBook)

More information about this series can be found at
https://novapublishers.com/product-category/series/new-developments-in-medical-research/

Stephen E. Bradley
Editor

Leptin and its Role in Health and Disease

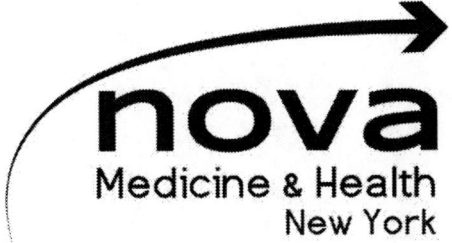

Copyright © 2024 by Nova Science Publishers, Inc.

All rights reserved. No part of this book may be reproduced, stored in a retrieval system or transmitted in any form or by any means: electronic, electrostatic, magnetic, tape, mechanical photocopying, recording or otherwise without the written permission of the Publisher.

We have partnered with Copyright Clearance Center to make it easy for you to obtain permissions to reuse content from this publication. Please visit copyright.com and search by Title, ISBN, or ISSN.

For further questions about using the service on copyright.com, please contact:

	Copyright Clearance Center	
Phone: +1-(978) 750-8400	Fax: +1-(978) 750-4470	E-mail: info@copyright.com

NOTICE TO THE READER

The Publisher has taken reasonable care in the preparation of this book but makes no expressed or implied warranty of any kind and assumes no responsibility for any errors or omissions. No liability is assumed for incidental or consequential damages in connection with or arising out of information contained in this book. The Publisher shall not be liable for any special, consequential, or exemplary damages resulting, in whole or in part, from the readers' use of, or reliance upon, this material. Any parts of this book based on government reports are so indicated and copyright is claimed for those parts to the extent applicable to compilations of such works.

Independent verification should be sought for any data, advice or recommendations contained in this book. In addition, no responsibility is assumed by the Publisher for any injury and/or damage to persons or property arising from any methods, products, instructions, ideas or otherwise contained in this publication.

This publication is designed to provide accurate and authoritative information with regards to the subject matter covered herein. It is sold with the clear understanding that the Publisher is not engaged in rendering legal or any other professional services. If legal or any other expert assistance is required, the services of a competent person should be sought. FROM A DECLARATION OF PARTICIPANTS JOINTLY ADOPTED BY A COMMITTEE OF THE AMERICAN BAR ASSOCIATION AND A COMMITTEE OF PUBLISHERS.

Library of Congress Cataloging-in-Publication Data

ISBN: 979-8-89113-274-0

Published by Nova Science Publishers, Inc. † New York

Contents

Preface		vii
Chapter 1	The Physiological and Pathophysiological Role of Leptin in Neurological and Behavioral Disorders	1
	Hayriye Soytürk, Ümit Kılıç and Ayşegül Yıldız	
Chapter 2	The Role of Leptin as a Biochemical Marker in Health and Disease	29
	Hadi Karimkhani	
Chapter 3	The Effects of Leptin on the Cardiovascular System	59
	Ümit Kılıç, Hayriye Soytürk, Eylem Suveren and Ayşegül Yıldız	
Chapter 4	Leptin in Reproductive Health and Disease	81
	D. G. Kishor Kumar, Ayushi Vaidhya, C. L. Madhu, Manjit Panigrahi, T. U. Singh, Dinesh Kumar and Subhashree Parida	
Chapter 5	The Role of Leptin in Diabetes and Its Complications	109
	Xiaoyu Xu, Yigang Feng, Cheng Zhang, Ning Wang and Yibin Feng	
Chapter 6	The Role of Leptin in Nutrition and Cancer	125
	Hasan Gencoglu and Kazim Sahin	
Chapter 7	A Molecular Overview of Leptin in Several Pathological Conditions	141
	Muge Atis Ceylan and Hilal Eren Gozel	
Index		161

Preface

This book contains seven chapters that detail leptin and its role in health and disease. Chapter One discusses many features of leptin and emphasizes the significance of future research to better understand leptin's involvement in neurological and behavioral disease causes and therapy. Chapter Two details the role of leptin as a biochemical marker. Chapter Three presents the consequences of hyperleptinemia caused by high leptin serum levels and leptin receptor resistance in obesity on renal, cardiac, vascular, and sympathetic nervous system function. The objective of Chapter Four is to shed light on the reproductive functions of leptin and its role in altered reproductive physiology. Chapter Five discusses the role of leptin in the pathogenesis and progression of diabetes and diabetic complications. Chapter Six summarizes the current understanding of the role of leptin in nutrition and cancer. Lastly, Chapter Seven provides a comprehensive review on the importance of leptin during different pathological conditions.

Chapter 1

The Physiological and Pathophysiological Role of Leptin in Neurological and Behavioral Disorders

Hayriye Soytürk[1],*, PhD
Ümit Kılıç[2], PhD
and Ayşegül Yıldız[3], PhD

[1]Bolu Abant Izzet Baysal University,
Institute of Graduate Studies Interdisciplinary Neuroscience, Bolu, Turkey
[2]Duzce University Vocational School of Health Services, Duzce, Turkey
[3]Bolu Abant Izzet Baysal University, Medical School,
Department of Physiology Bolu, Turkey

Abstract

Many factors can impact behavioral problems, including genetic, physiological, structural, and psychological factors. The genesis of behavioral disorders is influenced by several elements as a result of this complicated relationship. Because hormones are so tightly linked to the brain and nervous system, behavioral issues might be hormonal. Because of receptor insensitivity, the number of hormones may drop or rise; the number of receptors may alter; and mutations may develop. Leptin is a hormone that is generated mostly by fatty tissue, although it can also be produced by the placenta, skeletal muscle, stomach, mammary epithelium, and brain tissue. The hypothalamus, one of the body's most important organs, regulates the hormone leptin's physiological role and systemic effect. The leptin hormone inhibits appetite while increasing energy consumption in the hypothalamus arcuate nucleus. Leptin has

---

* Corresponding Author's Email: hayriyesoyturk1@gmail.com.

In: Leptin and its Role in Health and Disease
Editor: Stephen E. Bradley
ISBN: 979-8-89113-274-0
© 2024 Nova Science Publishers, Inc.

been shown to have both peripheral and central effects, interacting with the endocrine system and hence possibly impacting behavior. Eating disorders, schizophrenia, sleep, sexual behavior, depression, anxiety, anorexia nervosa, bipolar illness, borderline personality disorder, and alcohol use disorders have all been connected to leptin. According to studies, leptin has been linked to several behavioral illnesses, including depression. Furthermore, the interaction of antidepressants and antipsychotics with the hormone leptin has emerged as a new topic of research.

The role of leptin in neurological and behavioral diseases is emphasized in this book chapter. The chapter discusses many features of leptin and emphasizes the significance of future research to better understand leptin's involvement in disease causes and therapy.

Keywords: leptin, behavioral and neurological disorders

Introduction

Leptin, which is primarily produced and released by white adipose tissue, acts as an antiobesity agent by influencing its particular receptors in the hypothalamus, controlling the balance between energy intake and energy expenditure. Many factors influence the synthesis and secretion of leptin, which has been linked to a variety of functions including reproduction, hematopoiesis, gastrointestinal regulation, angiogenesis, sympathetic nervous system activation regulation, bone density determination, thermogenesis, and brain development.

Leptin regulates dietary behavior, regulates metabolic rate, activates the sympathetic nervous system, stimulates angiogenesis, regulates thermoregulation, and has an influence on growth and development (Lee GH. 1996).

Leptin, General Properties and Function

Zhang et al. (Zang et al. 1994) discovered leptin in 1994. Leptin is an adipocytokine with a molecular weight of 16 kDa and a total of 167 amino acids, 21 of which are signal peptides that are primarily released from adipose tissue. Although adipocytokines have molecular structures and cellular activities comparable to cytokines, they have physiological effects more akin to hormones (MacDougald OA, Auwerx J, 1998).

Leptin regulates the amount of body fat storage in various neuroendocrine systems, including the reproductive system (Fernandez-Fernandez R, 2006; Casanueva FF., 1999; Tena-Sempere M., 2007; Ahima RS, 2000; Mantzoros CS, 2011; Dardeno TA., 2010). While it was previously thought that Leptin was only synthesized in white adipose tissue, it has since been demonstrated that Leptin is also synthesized in brown adipose tissue, hypothalamus, pituitary gland, gastric epithelium, skeletal muscle, and syncytiotrophoblast (Auwerx and Staels). Aydin, S., 1998). Leptin is a hormone that controls energy intake and consumption in the brain, activates hypothalamic areas, regulates the hypothalamo-hypophyseal axis through numerous neuroendocrine processes, and participates in a variety of biological activities. In humans, it is encoded by the ob/ob gene, which is located on the long arm of chromosome 7 (7q31) (Zhang Y. 1994; Pelleymounter MA. 1994).

The liver, stomach, breast tissue, bone marrow, gut, ovary, testicles, skeletal muscle, stomach, and placenta all produce leptin (Meier and Gressner 2004). The action of free or protein-bound leptin is attributed to the free form of leptin. The bulk of leptin in serum in obese people is free (Meier and Gressner 2004). In rats, leptin binds to three serum macromolecules of roughly 85, 176, and 240 kDa, whereas in humans, it binds to two serum macromolecules of approximately 176 and 240 kDa. Binding proteins are hypothesized to be leptin receptors in a soluble form. The biological activity and half-life of leptin are regulated by leptin-binding protein.

Leptin has a circulation half-life of around 30 minutes and is released intermittently for about 2-3 hours after meals. It has a diurnal pattern, peaking in the early morning and troughing in the afternoon. Women have greater serum levels than males. This is explained by the fact that women have more adipose tissue and a greater rate of subcutaneous fat. In addition to energy balance, leptin is involved in neuroendocrine activities, immune system modulation, glucose, lipid, and bone metabolism (Aslan K. S. 2004).

A genetic mutation has been identified in mice that causes overeating, low energy expenditure, and an extremely obese phenotype. This gene was named Ob, and mice with this mutation were named Ob/Ob. Leptin is the product of the "ob/ob gene" and is also called the "ob protein." The product of the gene defective in ob/ob mice is called leptin and is derived from the Greek word 'leptos' meaning thin (Ahima RS, 2004).

A genetic mutation in mice has been uncovered that promotes overeating and poor energy expenditure, resulting in an excessively obese phenotype. Ob was given to this gene, and mice with this mutation were given the moniker Ob/Ob. Leptin is produced by the "ob/ob gene" and is also known as the "ob protein." The result of the faulty gene in ob/ob mice is termed leptin, which is derived from the Greek word 'leptos,' which means thin (Ahima RS, 2004).

Furthermore, Leptin is an adipokine that is generated insulin-dependently from white adipose tissue and triggers a pro-inflammatory response by boosting IL-6 and TNF-a production. Increased leptin levels, on the other hand, produce insulin resistance (Santoro A. 2015).

Because of the rise in adipose tissue caused by low leptin levels, it is considered that leptin is a hunger and weight gain hormone (Farooqi IS,2007; Rosenbaum M2002). Energy storage, food consumption, gender, age, physical activity, and glucose intake are all factors that influence leptin levels in the blood (O'Rahilly S.2014; Gruzdeva O,2019).

People with low or no leptin levels have been found to have deficiencies in reproductive development and function. Not only do leptin levels matter, but so do the quantity and function of receptors. Defective leptin signaling has been linked to early or late puberty, impairing fertility (Farooqi IS, O'Rahilly S, 2014; Roa J, Garcia-Galiano D, 2010).

Leptin has been linked to hunger metabolism and energy balance, and research has demonstrated that it is an effective anti-obesity agent with a feedback mechanism from adipocytes to the hypothalamus (Zhang et al. 1994).

Leptin Biosynthesis and Regulation

The number of adipocytes in the body is directly related to the control of leptin production and secretion. Leptin is linked to absolute fat mass as opposed to fat percentage or mass index. It has been observed that the quantity of leptin mRNA in adipose tissue is closely connected to the amount of leptin found in the blood (Bartness and Bamshad 1998; Baile et al. 2000). The majority of leptin secreted in the body comes from white adipose tissue and enters the circulation. Leptin is also generated by brain and gastrointestinal endocrine cells (Zhang Y, 2017). Structural leptin mRNA has been found in placental trophoblasts and amniotic cells, as well as certain tissues like bone and cartilage (Fantuzzi G. 2000). Leptin has a half-life of around 30 minutes in circulation and is released pulsatively 2-3 hours after meals (Aslan K. 2004). Leptin circulates in serum both free and attached to proteins (Zhang F. 2005). Internal organs such as the liver, particularly the kidneys, secrete leptin (Zeng et al. 1997).

Circulating leptin levels follow a 24-hour cycle. According to one study (Van Aggel Leijssen et al. 1999), leptin levels rise in the afternoon, peak after midnight, and then fall near daybreak. According to Goumenou et al. (2002), leptin has an appetite-reducing impact during sleep at night, which may be attributed to the influence of meals consumed during the day and hyperinsulinemia. In addition to the hormones leptin and thyroid, insulin-like growth factor (IGF) circulates bound to particular IGF-binding proteins (Sinha MK, 1996). The quantity of adipose tissue and the level of circulating leptin are positively associated (Considine RV, 1996).

Gender variations in circulating leptin concentration are evident. It is well known that estrogen activates leptin in women and increases leptin synthesis in subcutaneous adipose tissue, whereas testosterone suppresses leptin in males. As a result, women have three times the plasma leptin concentration per unit of fat mass as men. Ostlund RE Jr, 1996; Zhang F, 2005). Unlike humans, male rats have higher levels of leptin than females (Ahima RS., 2004).

It has been demonstrated that the level of circulating leptin rises in disorders like nutrition and obesity, but it falls in fasting. Fasting causes a drop in serum leptin levels, indicating that leptin production is controlled by variables other than body fat mass (Boden G., 1996). The size of adipocytes is another factor that influences the amount of circulating leptin. Leptin levels are higher in larger adipocytes than in tiny adipocytes (van Swieten MM., 2014; Kolaczynski JW., 1996).

Other than fasting, exposure to colds, catecholamines, and melatonin lowers leptin levels while increasing insulin levels (Wang Y., 2014). On the other side, steroid hormones raise Leptin levels. Furthermore, glucocorticoids have been shown to enhance leptin mRNA levels as well as release (Leal-Cerro A. 2001; Slieker LJ, 1996). Leptin expression is increased by Cortico hormone (CRH) (Fahlbusch FB., 2012). Leptin secretion is increased by oxytocin (Assinder SJ., 2021). Thyroid hormones inhibit leptin release (Escobar-Morreale HF, 1997). Catecholamines have been shown to decrease leptin release from differentiated human adipocytes via beta 1 and beta 2 adrenergic receptors (Boucsein A, 2021).

Leptin is also useful in the production and absorption of fatty acids. In vitro studies have demonstrated that leptin suppresses the production of acetyl-CoA carboxylase and fatty acid synthetase enzymes, which restrict fatty acid synthesis. Malonyl CoA is reduced when acetyl-CoA carboxylase is inhibited. As a result, when fatty acid absorption rises, so does oxidation. Leptin enhances the expression of lipoprotein lipase in brown adipose tissue (Scarpace and Matheny 1998; SiegristKaiser et al. 1997).

Metabolic hormones have a significant impact on physiological events such as lipogenesis and lipolysis, as well as reproduction and growth. Experiments have shown that leptin is important among metabolic hormones such as insulin and growth hormone. Body weight equilibrium is achieved by interactions between peripheral tissue and the hypothalamus via the hormone leptin (Baile et al. 2000).

Leptin Receptors

The leptin receptor belongs to the extended class I cytokine receptor family, which has six variations. Ob-Ra and Ob-Rb are the names of these receptors. Ob-Rc and Ob-Rd Ob-Rf and Ob-Re. Leptin receptor short forms, Ob-Ra, Ob-Rc, Ob-Rd, and Ob-Rf, are important for leptin trafficking across the blood-brain barrier since they are expressed largely in the choroid plexus, vascular endothelium, and peripheral tissues (Van Swieten MM, 2014). Leptin signaling is controlled by the long form of the Leptin Receptor (Ob-Rb). Ob-Rb, the long version of the leptin receptor, is prevalent in ARC, VMN, DMN, and LHA (Van Swieten MM, 2014).

Leptin's weight-regulating actions are mediated by OB-Rb in the hypothalamus. OB-Rb is also found in a variety of peripheral tissues. Leukemia cells, in particular endothelial cells, platelets, T lymphocytes, the yolk sac, and the fetal liver, express OB-Rb (Fantuzzi G, 2000).

Leptin signaling, like that of class I cytokine receptors, is assumed to be predominantly mediated by the Janus kinase/signal converter and activator of transcription (JAK-STAT). Only the long receptor JAK/STAT includes intracellular patterns essential for signal transduction pathway activation (Ahima RS, 2004). The JAK/STAT signal transduction system is activated by the long form of the leptin receptor, which reduces the activity of orexigenic peptides in ARC (Leshan RL. 2006).

Leptin's Physiological Function and Mechanism

Leptin primarily affects the central nervous system. Leptin is actively carried to the brain, where it primarily binds to the long form of its receptor in the arcuate nucleus (ARC) (Güldemir, H., 2018). Leptin possesses anorexigenic properties in the hypothalamus, particularly in the ARC (Balthasar N. 2004; van Swieten MM., 2014).

Leptin targets, orexigenic NPY/AgRP neurons, and anorexigenic CART/POMC neurons are all found in the ARC. While leptin inhibits and decreases the release of NPY/AgRP neurons, it stimulates POMC and CART gene expression and activates POMC/CART neurons (Münzberg H., 2015). Leptin's anorexigenic function is primarily accomplished by decreasing the signal of NPY, an orexigenic peptide, in the ARC-PVN axis (Kalra SP., 2008). Leptin causes POMC neurons to depolarize. When POMC neurons are stimulated, the amount of α-MSH released rises (Baldini G., 2019).

α-MSH produced by POMC neurons binds to MC4R expressed in PVN, signifying a reduction in energy intake and appetite suppression (Baldini G. 2019). Leptin enhances action potential frequency in anorexigenic POMC neurons via two mechanisms: depolarization via a nonspecific cation channel and decreased inhibition by nearby orexigenic NPY/GABA neurons. Furthermore, melanocortin peptides block this circuit by themselves (Cowley MA., 2001).

Leptin activates signal transducer and activator of transcription 3 (STAT3) in both POMC and NPY neurons, which is required for leptin's impact on ARC neurons. POMC transcription is induced by leptin activation of STAT3. Obesity is caused by a loss of leptin's capacity to activate STAT3 (Morrison CD., 2009). Leptin works on inhibitory collaterals that project NPY to POMC neurons, reducing GABA and NPY release from terminals (van Swieten MM.,) Leptin has metabolic effects in the central nervous system as well as peripheral organs (lung, liver, heart, pancreas, kidney, adrenal glands, ovary, uterus, testis, and so on) that interact with receptors (Goumenou et al. 2002).

Leptin produces hyperpolarization by activating an ATP-sensitive potassium channel. The hypothalamus is the primary location of action for leptin receptors. It is located in the hypothalamus region, which is related to reproduction, growth regulation, and hunger (Yu et al. 1997; Jin et al. 1999).

Leptin is also defined as a fat cell-derived signaling factor. After interacting with its receptors, it stimulates responses such as the control of body weight and energy expenditure, as well as plays a role in reproduction and neuroendocrine signaling. It plays an important role in the control of the onset of puberty, insulin resistance, and regulation of hypothalamic-pituitary functions, as well as participating in the cardiovascular system and urinary system (Goumenou et al. 2002).

Gender is one element that influences leptin levels. Females have greater leptin levels than men, depending on body mass index, total adipose tissue, body fat ratio, and age (Schwartz and Seeley 1997).

This condition is assumed to be produced by the fact that the fat ratio is higher and the distribution is different in females, the leptin blood levels are higher, and testosterone suppresses leptin levels in men (Himms-Hagen 1999).

Although leptin is a fat storage regulator, it also plays an essential function in animal adaptation to over- and under-nutrition. While animals with inadequate and imbalanced meals have a quick fall in plasma leptin levels, they also have a decrease in reproduction, thyroid activity, protein synthesis, and energy expenditure (Chelikani et al. 2004).

According to human research, insulin has little immediate effect on boosting leptin concentration, and leptin concentration increases after high insulin levels (D'Adamo et al. 1998).

Continuous leptin treatment enhances insulin sensitivity in vivo, although leptin exposure in vitro has little effect on glucose transport in the presence or absence of insulin (Zierath et al. 1998).

Glucocorticoids have been shown to boost leptin production whereas adrenergic stimulation reduces it. Chronic leptin injection increases GLUT4 levels and glucose utilization in brown adipose tissue while decreasing GLUT4 levels and glucose absorption in white adipose tissue. This application improves the sensitivity of the liver tissue to insulin and insulin-stimulated glycogen production. When varied amounts of leptin are given to experimental animals, glucose homeostasis is improved (Fruhbeck et al. 1998).

Ob/ob mice were shown to have decreased food intake and increased energy expenditure after receiving daily leptin injections, resulting in considerable weight reduction (Kim 1996).

Although there are no substantial changes in body weight during fasting, it has been demonstrated that blood leptin levels decline in tandem with glucose and insulin levels (Morton et al. 1999).

The Physiological Role of Leptin in the Central Nervous System

According to reports, leptin has receptors in both the brain and peripheral tissues and regulates nutrition, thermogenesis, the immune system, reproduction, bone density, brain development, hemodynamics, respiration, sympathetic nerve activity, and insulin-related functions in the liver via these receptors. The central nervous system handles the majority of these functions. Leptin's effects on the central nervous system are significantly more prevalent. It has been discovered that leptin shortage causes a reduction in brain weight as well as structural changes in neurons. Little is known about leptin's brain entrance. Leptin must travel through the Blood Cerebrospinal Fluid (BCSF) and/or the Blood-Brain Barrier (BBB) to reach various areas of the brain. According to certain research, the concentration of Leptin in cerebral fluid is inversely linked to the plasma concentration of Leptin (Schwartz MW. 1996). Because of this trait, men have larger levels of leptin in their cerebral fluid than women (Koistinen HA. 1998). Aside from this, another factor influencing Leptin content in cerebrospinal fluid is transport system saturation (Banks WA. 1996).

Recent in situ brain perfusion investigations have identified and characterized the kinetic characteristics of transporters involved in the transport of leptin from both BCSF and BBB. Although short-form receptors are thought to be carriers, it is also possible that the carriers have a different origin. The fact that cold Leptin treatment cannot entirely prevent brain Leptin absorption (ob/ob and db/db mice) shows that the receptors and transporters may have distinct origins and that a saturable/non-saturable dual transport system exists (Nam S-Y. 2001).

The BBB transports leptin to all parts of the brain. However, this transport rate reflects regional variations in the brain, because the levels of leptin in each brain area varies. The hypothalamus is the brain area with the greatest rate of leptin absorption. In contrast, the cerebral cortex has the slowest leptin absorption. Leptin transport to the brain is not proportional to serum Leptin levels (Campfield LA. 1995). Rapid transfer increases at low blood Leptin levels but not at the same pace as serum Leptin levels rise. This suggests that the Leptin transporters are saturated. The saturation found in leptin transport in the brain varies by brain region. This shows that when serum Leptin levels rise from low to high, some brain regions exhibit reduced transport sensitivity. While serum Leptin levels are high, the pons and medulla have the highest rate of transport (Campfield LA. 1995).

The hypothalamus has the slowest transport rate, which is lower than the brain's average transport rate. As a result, the serum Leptin level that initiates transport in each area of the brain varies. Furthermore, if the various actions of leptin occur through distinct brain areas, the optimal serum leptin levels will change for each impact of leptin (Schwartz MW., 1996).

Data collected thus far show that leptin resistance is induced by abnormalities in both the BBB transporters and the central nervous system receptors. Obesity is caused primarily by abnormalities in the transport of serum leptin from the BBB, according to findings from human and animal trials (Banks WA. 2001).

Obese Zucker rats, obese Koletsky rats, diet-enhanced LEW rats, and mice with maturation obesity have been shown to have decreased or missing leptin transport from the BBB. Although obese mice have three times the serum Leptin levels of normal mice, their leptin transport is three times lower. This finding indicates that the BBB transport issue is to blame for almost all leptin resistance. Similar studies in humans have demonstrated that transport system diseases are far more significant than Leptin receptor problems in the CNS (Banks WA., 2002).

Leptin transit and saturation vary by brain region. There are significant variances in the maximal quantity of Leptin delivered to the central nervous system across different areas of the brain. The hypothalamus has the highest degree of leptin transport, whereas the cerebral cortex has the lowest (Zlokovic BV. 2000).

The Relationship of Leptin with Neurological Diseases

Leptin expression levels and signaling pathways have been linked to neurological illnesses such as Parkinson's disease, epilepsy, ischemic stroke, migraine, cognitive decline, and dementia (Warren MW. 2012; Markaki E. 2012; Kantorova E. 2011). Parkinson's disease is a neurological disorder. The pathophysiology of Parkinson's disease, one of the most prevalent neurodegenerative disorders, is thought to be caused by a decline in the number of dopaminergic neurons in the substantia nigra (Randhawa BK. 2013; Schapira AH. 2013).

Leptin and Epilepsy

Leptin has been shown to have a proconvulsant action when combined with NMDA and kainate activation (Lynch JJ 2010). According to Aslan A. (2010), leptin, which enhances the frequency of penicillin-induced epileptic activity, does so via NO. However, Aslan A. (2009) claims that ghrelin, which has the opposite effect of leptin, also has an inhibitory impact on penicillin-induced epileptiform activity. According to a research examining the regulation and function of astrocytic leptin receptors in vitro and in vivo investigations, leptin signaling protects against seizures in astrocytes and partially mediates glutamate toxicity reduction (Jayaram B. 2013).

Leptin and Cerebral Ischemia

It has been reported that leptin has neuroprotective effects in vitro and in vivo experimental models by stimulating neurogenesis and angiogenesis against neuronal damage caused by ischemic stroke and that it may be an effective candidate for stroke treatment (Zhang F. 2007; Avraham Y. 2011; Avraham Y. 2013). According to Zhang et al. leptin protects against brain ischemia via activating the PI3K/Akt signaling pathway (Zhang J. 2013).

Leptin and Migraine

The growing interest in the headache and migraine groups in recent years is because this hormone is present in larger levels in obese women, and it is well known that these two categories are more affected by headache and migraine sickness. This is owing to the possibility that it is a factor. It was discovered in mouse research that injecting Leptin increases pain sensitivity while administering ibuprofen decreases Leptin levels (Hirfanoglu T. 2009; Peterlin BL. 2009).

Studies investigating the association between leptin levels and migraine, on the other hand, have shown inconclusive results. Leptin and insulin levels were examined in non-obese migraine sufferers and a healthy control group in a recent Austrian research. Insulin and leptin levels were discovered to be connected. Researchers believe that Leptin resistance may play a role in the pathogenesis (Bernecker. 2010).

In another study, the Leptin level was found to be higher than the basal values after prophylactic treatment in migraine patients, which was interpreted as the basal level of leptin being low, and the elevated levels of Leptin, which caused an increase in inflammatory and pain sensitization, may have caused Leptin resistance. The rise in leptin level did not spare the patient from migraine in this trial; the frequency and length of attacks remained the same, but the degree of pain was reduced (Hirfanoglu T. 2009; Peterlin BL. 2009).

It can be detected in both the blood and the cerebrospinal fluid. It uses a saturable transport method to traverse the blood-brain barrier. Leptin receptors are members of the cytokine class I receptor family and are present throughout the body. Leptin receptors are mostly found in the hypothalamus, but they also operate in the pituitary, brain stem, amygdala, thalamus, gyrus dentatus, and cerebellum. The obese gene is responsible for its expression. It regulates lipid and glucose homeostasis, the immune system, inflammation, and bone physiology. In arcuate neurons, there are two primary leptin-responsive groups: orexigenic (AgRP-NPY) and anorexigenic (CART (cocaine amphetamine-related transcript) -POMC (proopiomelanocortin) (McGregor G. 2017). Leptin suppresses the orexigenic group while activating the anorexigenic group. MAP2 is a somatodendritic marker found in ObRS + somatodendritic areas. Obrs are activated by Class 1 cytokines and provide leptin-dependent JAK2 phosphorylation through STAT, transcription factor, Ras MAPK, and PI-3 Kinase. In POMC-expressing hypothalamus neurons, ObR activation phosphorylates STAT3. It maintains homeostasis and energy balance. STAT3 activation promotes dentate gyrus regeneration as well as leptin neuroprotection, whereas ERK signaling promotes hypothalamic feeding. Leptin also stimulates the mTOR and Fox01 signaling pathways (McGregor G. 2017). Lipodystrophy, hypothalamic amenorrhea, and congenital leptin insufficiency are all caused by a mutation in the leptin gene. Increased insulin resistance, hyperlipidemia, endocrine diseases, morbid obesity, and cognitive impairment can all result from a lack of it. Leptin replacement stimulates the appetite, satiety, and reward centers of the brain. In fMRI investigations, leptin supplementation blocked the hunger regions of the insula, parietal, and temporal cortex while activating the satiety areas of the prefrontal and frontal cortex (McGregor G. 2017). Leptin receptors come in both short and long versions. The long form is more frequent in the hypothalamus, whereas the short form is present throughout the body. The short form is in charge of leptin's peripheral actions (Houseknecht KL. 1998).

Relationship between Leptin, Cognition and Alzheimer's

Leptin is involved in hippocampus neuron synaptic function, glial maturation, ischemic damage mitigation in temporary ischemia, and mitochondrial membrane stability (Ülker M. 2018). There is a reduction in cognition and memory when it is deficient or resistant. Leptin reduces A buildup, presenilin transcription, and tau phosphorylation by lowering beta-secretase activity, promotes ApoE-dependent amyloid absorption, and aids in beta-amyloid clearance by binding to the megalin/lrp2 receptor complex (engaged in beta-amyloid endocytosis) S. Kamohara, 1997; It suppresses tau phosphorylation and the creation of neurofibrillary tangles while also combating apoptotic cell death and contributing to hippocampus progenitor cell proliferation by inhibiting the GSK-3B enzyme. It accomplishes this by activating STAT) (S. Kamohara, 1997).

As a result, it enhances learning and memory performance. Leptin response and STAT 3 activation diminish with brain aging. NMDA receptors in hippocampal synapses activate leptin target leptin Ca2+ influx and boost NMDA receptor activity via STP-LTP conversion, (Shimabukuro M. 1997). Leptin-dependent LTP promotes AMPA receptor entrance into synapses. The PI3 kinase must be activated for LTP to occur. As a result, the activity of CA1-CA3 neurons at hippocampal synapses rises (Frühbeck G. 2001; Matthew J. McGuire. 2016).

Leptin Signaling in the Hippocampus Leptin stimulates the PI3K/AKT, JAK-STAT, and AMK/SIRT pathways in the hippocampus, the BACE 1 enzyme is down-regulated, A synthesis and clearance reduce, and tau phosphorylation lowers. STAT3 phosphorylation is stimulated by leptin receptors. Leptin suppresses tau hyperphosphorylation via PI3K and AKT activation. It inhibits GSK3-B through AMPK and decreases A deposit deposition. PGC-1 also has a BACE1 inhibition and An accumulation prevention effect (S. J. Greco. 2011).

Leptin lowers glutamate toxicity, promotes neurotrophic factor (BDNF) production, inhibits apoptotic enzymes, promotes the development of oligodendroglia, and boosts synaptic transmission. The table below summarizes the putative effects of leptin in the brain on the development of Alzheimer's type dementia (G. Paz Filho. 2010).

According to studies, a higher BMI value is connected with greater cognitive function. This is explained by the protective impact of leptin on the neurological system, which is associated with increased body fat (And Hudetz JA. 2011).

Leptin replacement has been demonstrated to enhance gray matter volume in the cerebellum, inferior parietal, and anterior cingulate gyrus in leptin-deficient people. In fMRI studies, leptin supplementation blocked the hunger centers insula, parietal, and temporal cortex, while activating the satiety regions prefrontal and frontal cortex. Reduced LTP and synaptic activity of hippocampal CA1 neurons have been found in animal models of hereditary leptin insufficiency and receptor resistance (Matochik J. A. 2005).

The hippocampus leptin response is known to decline with age. People with Alzheimer's disease who have high leptin levels in their CSF may develop neuronal leptin resistance. Hippocampal LepRb levels were shown to be reduced in postmortem AD brains. According to one theory, neurofibrillary tangles inhibit the leptin receptor from accessing circulating leptin in the brain, causing leptin levels in neurons in CSF to rise and resistance to develop. Circadian rhythm disruption has been linked to hypothalamus involvement in Alzheimer's disease (Matthew J. McGuire.2016).

Association of Leptin with Psychiatric Disorders

Apart from the fact that leptin has many peripheral and central effects, interacts with the endocrine system, opens the door to new research, and plays a role in obesity, diabetes, appetite, thermogenesis, immune system, and reproduction; it has also led to research on many psychiatric conditions such as sleep, sexual behavior, impulsivity, depression, anxiety, anorexia nervosa, bipolar disorder, borderline personality disorder, weight changes due to psychotropic Many research have been conducted to investigate its function in mental illnesses such as depression.

Depression and Leptin

According to Lu X. (2006), the hippocampus is a region that mediates leptin's antidepressant-like effect. Garza et al. discovered that prolonged leptin administration decreased stress-induced hippocampus neurogenesis and depression-like behaviors in rats subjected to unpredictable chronic mild stress (CUMS) (Garza JC. 2012). Depression-like behaviors are produced in rat models following CUMS treatment, as are blood leptin levels and hypothalamic leptin receptor mRNA expression (Ge JF. 2013). As a consequence, it is recognized that leptin, which is known to play an active part in a variety of physiological and physiopathological processes, is a hormone that should be addressed in the treatment and prognosis of a variety of diseases, including neurological and psychiatric disorders.

Leptin and Eating Disorders

According to the research, leptin levels vary in eating disorders such as Anorexia nervosa (AN) and Bulimia nervosa (BN) (Zupancic ML. 2011). Brewerton et al. found a link between leptin levels and body mass index, weight, and average body weight percentage in AN and BN patients (Brewerton TD. 2000). However, studies demonstrate that BN patients have lower leptin levels than normal controls and that there is no significant difference in serum leptin levels between these patients and AN patients (Jimerson DC. 2000; Monteleone P. 2002).

Anorexia nervosa (AN) is a condition of various endocrine problems marked by intense hunger and weight loss with uncertain causative reasons. In terms of body fat ratio, leptin levels were lower in AN patients (M. Haluzik. 1990).

While blood lipid, total protein, albumin, and albumin concentrations do not alter throughout the recovery period in AN patients, serum leptin levels do. This shows that leptin is a sensitive measure for AN patients' nutritional state (M. Haluzik. 1999; C. Mantzoros. 1997).

When serum leptin levels in female AN patients and healthy controls were compared, leptin levels were found to be significantly lower in the control group, and it was stated that low leptin levels may be associated with amenorrhea and a decreased metabolic rate in the disease (Hebebrand J. 1997).

Leptin and soluble leptin receptors were studied in 133 women with AN, bulimia nervosa (BN), obesity with binge eating episodes, and obese and healthy women without binge eating episodes. Obese women with or without binge eating episodes were shown to have a greater risk. Furthermore, soluble leptin receptors were shown to be abundant in AN and BN but absent in others (P. Monteleone. 2002). The fact that leptin levels are low, particularly in AN patients, and that the patient improves with weight gain following therapy shows that it may be an essential signal in the disease's progression (P. Monteleone. 2002).

Mood Disorders and Leptin

Studies on mood disorders are an essential component of leptin research. Several earlier research have found a link between blood cholesterol levels and mental problems. There have been studies that show low and high blood cholesterol levels in depression, as well as ones that show low cholesterol levels in mania (SN. Ghaemi, 2000).

Leptin has also been linked to the neuroendocrine system and cholesterol, as well as sleep, mobility, sexual behavior, and impulsive conduct. They discovered a negative link between YMRS and serum leptin and cholesterol levels, as well as a positive correlation between mean cholesterol and leptin levels (Atmaca M. 2002).

He investigated serum leptin levels and their nocturnal changes in depressed patients and discovered that serum leptin levels were associated with BMI in normal healthy individuals but not in depressed patients and that leptin secretion was impaired in depressive disorder (Antonijevic IA. 1998).

While blood leptin levels in female depression patients were found to be considerably higher than in healthy women, no significant difference was detected in males. They blamed central obesity and hypercortisolism arising from omental adipose tissue for the considerably higher leptin levels in both healthy and depressed women compared to men (RT Rubin, 2002).

Some leptin research looks at the association between suicide attempts and leptin. Low cholesterol levels have been linked to the severity of suicide and the manner of suicide (Lester D. 2002).

Schizophrenia and Leptin

Although leptin levels are favorably connected with schizophrenia symptoms, there is no association between leptin with neurocognitive or negative symptoms (Takayanagi Y. 2013). Many studies have indicated that leptin has a role in antipsychotic therapy and weight gain pathways (Herrán A. 2001; Pea R. 2008). According to several research, blood leptin levels increase following atypical antipsychotic therapy in individuals with schizophrenia, and leptin levels are shown to be high regardless of body mass index (Panariello F. 2012).

Conclusion

Leptin is a hormone that is generated mostly by fatty tissue, although it can also be produced by the placenta, skeletal muscle, stomach, mammary epithelium, and brain tissue. The hypothalamus, one of the body's most important organs, regulates the hormone leptin's physiological role and systemic effect. The leptin hormone inhibits appetite while increasing energy consumption in the hypothalamus arcuate nucleus. Leptin has been shown to have both peripheral and central effects, interacting with the endocrine system and hence possibly impacting behavior. Eating disorders, schizophrenia, sleep, sexual behavior, depression, anxiety, anorexia nervosa, bipolar illness, borderline personality disorder, and alcohol use disorders have all been connected to leptin. According to studies, leptin has been linked to several behavioral illnesses, including depression. Furthermore, the interaction of antidepressants and antipsychotics with the hormone leptin has emerged as a new topic of research.

As the prevalence of neurodegenerative disorders and mood disorders has increased in recent years, it is important to investigate the cellular and molecular mechanisms of these diseases. In recent studies, the antidepressant effects of leptin have been observed. It is an inevitable problem that neurological diseases and metabolic abnormalities can share overlapping brain circuits that combine homeostatic and regulatory responses and genetic susceptibility factors. Yet growing evidence suggests that leptin has a potential effect in reversing Alzheimer's symptoms. The effect of leptin may be based on a mechanism that increases the activation of neurons in the hippocampus, decreases amyloid-β and tau levels, and modulates microglia. Leptin appears to have neuroprotective effects on neurodegenerative disorders. More experimental and clinical research is needed to understand the relationship between leptin and neurological diseases.

References

Ahima RS, Dushay J, Flier SN, Prabakaran D, Flier JS. 1997. "Leptin accelerates the onset of puberty in. normal female mice." *J Clin Invest* 99:391–5.

Ahima RS, Osei SY. 2004. "Leptin signaling." *Physiol Behav* 81:223-41.

Ahima RS, Saper CB, Flier JS, Elmquist JK. 2000. "Leptin regulation of neuroendocrine systems." *Front Neuroendocrinol* 21: 263–307.

Antonijevic IA, Murck H, Frieboes RM, Horn R, Brabant G, Steiger A. 1998. "Elevated nocturnal profiles of serum leptin in patients with depression." *J Psychiatr Res.* Nov-Dec;32(6):403-10. doi: 10.1016/s0022-3956(98)00032-6. PMID: 9844957.

Arıkan Ş. 2013. Üniversite öğrencilerinin vücut ağırlığı, vücut kitle indeksi, plazma büyüme hormonu, ghrelin, leptin düzeyleri ve dayanıklılık antrenmanı arasındaki ilişkiler. *Selçuk Üniversitesi Sağlık Bilimleri Enstitüsü.*

Aslan A, Yildirim M, Ayyildiz M, Güven A, Agar E. 2009. The role of nitric oxide in the inhibitory effect of ghrelin against penicillin-induced epileptiform activity in rat. *Neuropeptides* 43(4):295-302.

Aslan A, Yildirim M, Ayyildiz M, Güven A. Agar E. 2010. Interaction of leptin and nitric oxide pathway on penicillininduced epileptiform activity in rats. *Brain Res* 19;1321:117-24.

Aslan K SZ, Tokullugil AH. 2004. Multifonksiyonel Hormon: Leptin. *Uludağ Üniversitesi Tıp Fakültesi Dergisi*;30(2):113-118.

Atmaca M, Kuloglu M, Tezcan E, Gecici O, Ustundag B. 2002. Serum cholesterol and leptin levels in patients with borderline personality disorder, Neuropsychobiology 45(4):167-71.

Atmaca M, Kuloglu M, Tezcan E, Ustundag B, Bayik Y. 2002. Serum leptin and cholesterol levels in patients with bipolar disorder. *Neuropsychobiology* 46(4):176-9. doi: 10.1159/000067809. PMID: 12566933.

Atmaca M, Kuloglu M, Tezcan E, Ustundag B. 2002. Weight gain and serum leptin levels in patients on lithium treatment. *Neuropsychobiology* 46(2):67-9. doi: 10.1159/000065414. PMID: 12378122.

Auwerx J, Staels B (1998). Leptin. *The Lancet* 351, 737-742.

Avraham Y, Davidi N, Lassri V, Vorobiev, L, Kabesa, M, Chernoguz, D, Berry, E, Leker, RR 2011. Leptin induces neuroprotection neurogenesis and angiogenesis after stroke. *Curr Neurovasc Res.* 8(4):313-22.

Avraham Y, Dayan M, Lassri V, Vorobiev, L, Davidi, N, Chernoguz, D, Berry, E, & Leker, RR. 2013. Delayed leptin administration after stroke induces neurogenesis and angiogenesis. *J Neurosci Res* 91(2):187-95.

Aydın S. 2007. Ghrelin hormonunun kesfi: Arastırmaları ve klinik uygulamaları. *Türk biyokimya Dergisi* 32:76Á89.

Baile CA, Della-Fera MA, Martin RJ (2000). Regulation of metabolism and body fat mass by leptin. *Ann Rev Nutrition*, 20, 105-127.

Baldini G, Phelan KD (2019). The melanocortin pathway and control of appetiteprogress and therapeutic implications. *J Endocrinol* 241:1-33.

Balthasar N, Coppari R, McMinn J, Liu SM, Lee CE, Tang V, Kenny CD, McGovern RA, Chua SC Jr, Elmquist JK, Lowell BB (2004). Leptin receptor signaling in POMC neurons is required for normal body weight homeostasis. *Neuron* 42:983-91.

Banks WA, Coon AB, Robinson SM, Moinuddin A, Shultz JM, Nakaoke R, Morley, JE. 2004. Triglycerides induce leptin resistance at the blood-brain barrier. *Diabetes* 53(5):1253-60.

Banks WA, Kastin AJ, Huang W, Jaspan JB, Maness LM. 1996. Leptin enters the brainby a saturable system independent of insulin. *Peptides* 17(2):305-11.

Banks WA, Niehoff ML, Martin D, Farrell CL. 2002. Leptin transport across the blood–brain barrier of the Koletsky rat is not mediated by a product of the leptin receptor gene. *Brain research* 950 (1-2):130-6.

Banks WA. 2001. Leptin transport across the blood-brain barrier: implications for the cause and treatment of obesity. *Current pharmaceutical design* 7(2):125-33.

Bartness TJ, Bamshad M (1998). Innervation of mammalian white adipose tissue: implications for the regulation of total body fat. *Am J Physiol* 275, 1399-1411.

Baumgartner RN, Waters DL, Morley JE, Patrick, P, Montoya, GD, & Garry, PJ. 1999. Age-related changes in sex hormones affect the sex difference in serum leptin independently of changes in body fat. *Metabolism* 48: 378–384.

Benskey M, Lee KY, Parikh K, Lookingland KJ, Goudreau JL. 2013. Sustained resistance to acute MPTP toxicity by hypothalamic dopamine neurons following chronic neurotoxicant exposure is associated with sustained upregulation of parkin protein. *Neurotoxicology* 37:144- 53.

Bernecker C, Pailer S, Kieslinger P, Horejsi R, Möller R, Lechner A, Wallner-Blazek, M, Weiss, S, Fazekas, F, Truschnig-Wilders, M, & Gruber, HJ. 2010. GLP2 and leptin are associated with hyperinsulinemia in non-obese female migraineurs. *Cephalalgia* 30(11):1366-.

Bjorbaek C, Kahn BB. 2004. Leptin signaling in the central nervous system and the periphery. *Recent progress in hormone research* 59:305-32.

Boden G, Chen X, Mozzoli M, Ryan I. 1996. Effect of fasting on serum leptin in normal human subjects. *J Clin Endorinol Metab* 81: 3419- 23.

Boucsein A, Kamstra K, Tups A (2021). Central signalling cross talk between insulin and leptin in glucose and energy homeostasis. *J Neuroendocrinol* 33:e12944.

Brabant G, Horn R, Mayr M, Wurster U, Schnabel D, Heidenreich F. 2000. Free and protein bound leptin are distinct and independently controlled factors in energy regulation. *Diabetologia* 43; 438-42.

Brewerton TD, Lesem MD, Kennedy A, Garvey WT. 2000. Reduced plasma leptin concentrations in bulimia nervosa. *Psychoneuroendocrinology* 25(7):649-58.

Campfield LA, Smith FJ, Guisez Y, Devos R, Burn P. 1995. Recombinant mouse OB protein: evidence for a peripheral signal linking adiposity and central neural networks. *Science* 269(5223):546-9.

Casabiell X, Pineiro V, Vega F, De La Cruz, LF, Dieguez, C, Casanueva, FF. 2001. Leptin, reproduction and sex steroids. *Pituitary* 4:93-99.

Casanueva FF, Dieguez C. 1999. Neuroendocrine regulation and actions of leptin. *Front Neuroendocrinol* 20:317–63.

Castellano JM, Roa J, Luque RM, Dieguez, C, Aguilar, E, Pinilla, L, & Tena-Sempere, M. 2009. KiSS-1/kisspeptins and the metabolic control of reproduction: Physiologic roles and putative physiopathological implications. *Peptides* 30: 139– 45.

Chehab FF, Mounzih K, Lu R, Lim ME. 1997. Early onset of reproductive function in normal female mice treated with leptin. *Science* 275:88–90.

Chelikani PK, Ambrose JD, Keisler DH, Kennelly JJ. 2004. Effect of short term fasting on plasma concentrations of leptin and other hormones and metabolites in dairy cattle. Dom Anim *Endocrinol,* 26, 33-48.

Cheung CC, Thornton JE, Kuijper JL, Weigle, DS, Clifton, DK, & Steiner, RA. 1997. Leptin is a metabolic gate for the onset of puberty in the female rat. *Endocrinology* 138:855–8.

Considine RV, Sinha MK, Heiman ML, Kriauciunas A, Stephens TW, Nyce MR, Ohannesian JP, Marco CC, McKee LJ, Bauer TL, José F. Caro MD. 1996. Serum immunoreactive-leptin concentrations in normal-weight and obese humans. *N Engl J Med* 334:292-5.

Coşkun A. 2012. Yeme bozukluklarında moleküler mekanizmalar. *Bilim ve Teknik* 2:58-62.
Cowley MA, Smart JL, Rubinstein M, Cerdán MG, Diano S, Horvath TL, Cone RD, Low MJ. 2001. Leptin activates anorexigenic POMC neurons through a neural network in the arcuate nucleus. *Nature* 411:480-4.
Cusin I, Sainsbury A, Doyle P, Rohner-Jeanrenaud F, Jeanrenaud B. 1995. The ob gene and insulin, a relationship leading to clues to the understanding of obesity. *Diabetes* 44: 1467-70.
D'Adamo M, Buongiorno A, Maroccia E, Leonetti F, Barbetti F, Giaccari A, Zorretta D, Tamburrano G, Sbraccia P. 1998. Increased OB gene expression leads to elevated plasma leptin concentrations in patients with chronic primary hyperinsulinemia. *Diabetes* 47, 10, 625-9.
Dardeno TA, Chou SH, Moon HS, Chamberland, JP, Fiorenza, CG, & Mantzoros, CS. 2010. Leptin in human physiology and therapeutics. *Front Neuroendocrinol* 31:377–93.
Eckert ED, Pomeroy C, Raymond N, Kohler PF, Thuras P, Bowers CY. 1998. Leptin in anorexia nervosa. *J Clin Endocrinol Metab* 83:791-795.
Fantuzzi G, Faggioni R. 2000. Leptin in the regulation of immunity, inflammation, and hematopoiesis. *J Leukoc Biol* 68:437-46.
Farooqi IS, Bullmore E, Keogh J, Gillard J, O'Rahilly S, Fletcher PC. 2007. Leptin regulates striatal regions and human eating behavior. *Science*;317(5843):1355-.
Farooqi IS, Jebb SA, Langmack G, Lawrence, E, Cheetham, CH, Prentice, AM, Hughes, IA, McCamish, MA, & O'Rahilly, S. 1999. Effects of recombinant leptin therapy in a child with congenital leptin deficiency. *N Engl J Med*;341:879–84.
Farooqi IS, O'Rahilly S. 2014. 20 YEARS OF LEPTIN: Human disorders of leptin action. *J Endocrinol* 223:T63–70.
Fernandez-Fernandez R, Martini AC, Navarro VM, Castellano, JM, Dieguez, C, Aguilar, E, Pinilla, L, & Tena-Sempere, M. 2006. Novel signals for the integration of energy balance and reproduction. *Mol Cell Endocrinol* 254–255:127–32.
Filier JS. 1997. Leptin expression and action: new experimental pradigms. *Proc Nat Acad Sci* s. 94: 4242-4245.
Flier JS. 1995. The adipocyte: storage depot or node on the energy information superhighway? Cell 80: 15-8.
Frederich RC, Hamann A, Anderson S, Löllmann B, Lowell BB, Flier JS. 1995. Leptin levels reflect body lipid content in mice: evidence for diet-induced resistance to leptin action. *Nat Med* 1:1311- 4.
Friedman JM, Halaas JL. 1998. Leptin and the regulation of body weight in mammals. *Nature* 395; 763-770.
Friedman JM. 1997. Role of leptin and its receptors in the control of body weight. In: (Blum WF, Kiess W & Rascher W eds.) Leptin-the voice of adipose tissue. *Johann Ambrosius Barth Verlag, Germany* 3-22.
Frühbeck G, Gomez-Ambrosi J, Muruzabal FJ, Burrel MA. 2001. The adipocyte: a model for integration of endocrine and metabolic signalling in energy metabolism regulation. *Am J Physical Endocrine Metab* 280: E827-E847.

G Ying Li. 2000. Anorexia nevrosa: disordered feedbac regulation in the Growth Hormone –Insulin-like Growth factor 1 axix. *Dartmouth Undergraduate Journal of science* 2(2).
G. Paz Filho, M.-L. Wong, J. Licinio. 2010. The procognitive effects of leptin in the brain and their clinical implications. *The İnternational Journal Of Clinical Practice.* 64(13):1808-12.
Garza JC, Guo M, Zhang W, Lu XY. 2012. Leptin restores adult hippocampal neurogenesis in a chronic unpredictable stress model of depression and reverses glucocorticoid-induced inhibition of GSK-3β/β-catenin signaling. *Mol Psychiatry* 17(8):790-808.
Ge JF, Qi CC, Zhou JN. 2013. Imbalance of leptin pathway and hypothalamus synaptic plasticity markers are associated with stress-induceddepression in rats. *Behav Brain Res.* 15;249:38-43.
Ghaemi SN, Shields GS, Hegarty JD, Goodwin FK. 2000. Cholesterol levels in mood disorders: high or low? *Bipolar Disord.* Mar;2(1):60-4. doi: 10.1034/j.1399-5618.2000.020109.x. PMID: 11254022.
Gómez-Ambrosi J, Salvador J, Páramo JA, Orbe J, de Irala J, Diez-Caballero A, Gil, MJ, Clenfuegos, JA, & Frühbeck, G. Involvement of leptin in the association between percentage of body fat and cardiovascular risk factors. *Clinical biochemistry.* 2002;35(4):315-20.
Goumenou AG, Matalliotakis IM, Koumantakis GE, Panidis DK (2002). The role of leptin in fertility. *Eur J Obs & Gyn Reprod Biol*, 106, 118-124.
Greco, SJ, Hamzelou, A, Johnston, JM, Smith, MA, Ashford, JW, Tezapsidis, N, Leptin boosts cellular metabolism by activating AMPK the sirtuins to reduce tau phosphorylation and β-amyloid in neurons, *Biochem. Biophys. Res. Commun.* 14(2011):203-217.
Gruzdeva O, Borodkina D, Uchasova E, Dyleva Y, Barbarash O. Leptin resistance: underlying mechanisms and diagnosis. *Diabetes, metabolic syndrome and obesity: targets and therapy.* 2019;12:191.
Güldemir, H. (2018). Yüksek yağlı diyetin açlık-tokluk metabolizmasında görevli hormonlar ve nöropeptidler üzerine etkileri. *Sağlık Bilimleri Dergisi* 27, 239-344.
Guzik TJ, Mangalat D, Korbut R. Adipocytokines-novel link between inflammation and vascular function? *J Physiol Pharmacol*. 2006; 57: 505-528.
Haluzik M, Fieldler J, Nedvinkova J, Ceska R: Serum leptin concentrations in patients with combined, hyperlipidemia, relationships to serum lipids and lipoproteins. *Physiol Res* 1999;48:363-368.
Haluzík M, Papezová M, Nedvídková J, Kábrt J. Serum leptin levels in patients with anorexia nervosa before and after partial refeeding, relationships to serum lipids and biochemical nutritional parameters. *Physiol Res.* 1999;48(3):197-202. PMID: 10523055.
Hardie L, Trayhurn P, Abramovich D, & Fowler, P. Circulating leptin in women: a longitudinal study in the menstrual cycle and during pregnancy. *Clin Endocrinol* 1997; 47: 101–106.
Harvey J, Ashford MLJ. Leptin in the CNS: much more than a satiety signal. *Neuropharmacology* 2003; 44: 845–854.
Haynes WG, Sivitz WI, Morgan DA, Walsh SA, Mark AL. Sympathetic and cardiorenal actions of leptin. *Hypertension* 1997; 30: 619-623.

Hebebrand J, Blum WF, Barth N, Coners H, Englaro P, Juul A, Ziegler A, Warnke A, Rascher W, Remschmidt H. 1997. Leptin levels in patients with anorexia nervosa are reduced in the acute stage and elevated upon short-term weight restoration. *Mol Psychiatry* Jul;2(4):330-4. doi: 10.1038/sj.mp.4000282. PMID: 9246674.

Herrán A, García-Unzueta MT, Amado JA, de La Maza MT, Alvarez C, Vázquez-Barquero JL. 2001. Effects of long-term treatment with antipsychotics on serum leptin levels. *Br J Psychiatry*. 179:59-62.

Himms-Hagen J. 1999. Physiological roles of the leptin endocrine system: Differences between Mice and Humans. *Crit Rev Cl Lab Sci* 36, 6, 575- 655.

Hirfanoglu T, Serdaroglu A, Gulbahar O, Cansu A. 2009. Prophylactic drugs and cytokine and leptin levels in children with migraine. *Pediatric neurology*. 41(4): 281-7.

Houseknecht KL, Baile CA, Matteri RL, Spurlock ME. 1998. The Biology of Leptin: A Review. *J Anim Sci* 76: 1405-1420.

Houseknecht KL, Portocarrero CP. 1998. Leptin and its receptors: regulators of wholebody energy homeostasis. *Domest Anim Endocrin* 15, 457-475.

Jayaram B, Khan RS, Kastin AJ, Hsuchou H, Wu X, Pan W., Protective role of astrocytic leptin signaling against excitotoxicity, *J Mol Neurosci*. 2013;49(3):523-30.

Jimerson DC, Mantzoros C, Wolfe BE, Metzger ED. Decreased serum leptin in bulimia nervosa. J Clin Endocrinol Metab. 2000;85(12):4511-4.

Kalra SP (2008). Disruption in the leptin-NPY link underlies the pandemic of diabetes and metabolic syndrome: new therapeutic approaches. Nutrition 24:820-6.

Kamohara S, Burcelin R, Halaas JL, Friedman JM, Charron MJ. Acute stimulation of glucose metabolism in mice by leptin treatment. Nature 1997; 389: 374-7..

Kandi B. Investigation of osteopontin, apelin, leptin and adiponektin levels in patients with psoriazis and evaluate the relationship between the metabolic syndrome. 2011.

Kantorova E, Chomova M, Kurca, E, Sivak, S, Zelenak, K, Kucera, P, Galajda, P. Leptin, adiponectin and ghrelin, new potential mediators of ischemic stroke, *Neuro Endocrinol Lett*. 2011;32(5):716-21.

Karlsson C. 2000. Leptin-a slimmer's dream that crashed? *J Int F Clin Chem Lab Med*, 12, 1-9.

Kim KH. 1996. Scientists Sprint to Understand Fat-Busting Protein Leptin. *Purdue News*, 11.

Kitamura T. Forkhead protein FoxO1 mediates Agrp-dependent effects of leptin on food intake. *Nat Med*. 2006; 12(5): 534-40.

Koistinen HA, Karonen S-L, Iivanainen M, Koivisto VA. Circulating leptin has saturable transport into intrathecal space in humans. *European journal of clinical investigation*. 1998;28(11):894-7.

Lee GH, Proenza R, Montez JM, Carroll KM, Darvishzadch JG, Lee JL, Friedman, JM. Abnormal splicing of the leptin receptor in diabetic mice. *Nature* 1996; 39: 632-635.

Leshan RL, Björnholm M, Münzberg H, Myers MG Jr (2006). Leptin receptor signaling and action in the central nervous system. *Obesity* (Silver Spring) 5:208-212.

Lester D. Serum cholesterol levels and suicide: a meta-analysis. *Suicide Life Threat Behav*. 2002 Fall;32(3):333-46. doi: 10.1521/suli.32.3.333.22177. PMID: 12374479.

Li Hf, Zou Y, Xia Zz, Gao F, Feng Jh, Yang Cw. Effects of topiramate on weight and metabolism in children with epilepsy. *Acta Paediatrica*. 2009;98(9):1521-5.

Licinio J, Negrão AB, Mantzoros C, Kaklamani, V, Wong, ML, Bongiorno, PB, Negro, PP, Mulla, A, Veldhuis, JD, Cearnal, L, Flier, JS, Gold, PW. Sex differences in circulating human leptin pulse amplitude: clinical implications. *J Clin Endocrinol Metab* 1998; 83: 4140–4147.

Ligong Z, Jinjin Q, Chunfu C, Congcong L, Xiaojun D. Effect of obesity and leptin level on migraineurs. *Medical science monitor: international medical journal of experimental and clinical research*. 2015;21:3270.

Lu X, Kim C, Frazer A, Zhang W. Leptin: a potential novel antidepressant. *Proc Natl Acad Sci U S A* 2006; 103: 1593–8.

Lynch JJ 3rd, Shek EW, Castagné V, Mittelstadt SW. The proconvulsant effects of leptin on glutamate receptormediated seizures in mice. *Brain Res Bull*. 2010 29;82(1-2):99-103.

Ma Z, Gingerich RL, Santiago JV, Klein S, Smith CH, Landt M. Radioimmunoassay of leptin in human plasma. *Clin Chem* 1996, 42: 942- 6.

MacDougald OA, Burant CF. The rapidly expanding family of adipokines. *Cell metabolism*. 2007;6(3):159-61.

Magnia P, Vektor R, Pagano C, Calcagno A, Martini L, Motta M. Control of the expression of human neuropeptide Y by leptin : in vitro studies. *Peptides* 2001; 22: 415-420.

Mantzoros C, Flier JS, Lesem MD, Brewerton TD, Jimerson DC. Cerebrospinal fluid leptin in anorexia nervosa: correlation with nutritional status and potential role in resistance to weight gain. *J Clin Endocrinol Metab*. 1997 Jun;82(6):1845-51. doi: 10.1210/jcem.82.6.4006. PMID: 9177394.

Mantzoros CS, Magkos F, Brinkoetter M, Sienkiewicz, E, Dardeno, TA, Kim, SY, Hamnvik, OPR, & Koniaris, A. Leptin in human physiology and pathophysiology. *Am J Physiol Endocrinol Metab* 2011;301:E567–84.

Markaki E, Ellul J, Kefalopoulou Z, Trachani, E., Theodoropoulou, A., Kyriazopoulou, V., & Constantoyannis, C. The role of ghrelin, neuropeptide Y and leptin peptides in weight gain after deep brain stimulation for Parkinson's disease, *Stereotact Funct Neurosurg*. 2012;90(2):104-12.

Masdrakis VG, Papageorgiou C, Markianos M. Associations of plasma leptin to clinical manifestations in reproductive aged female patients with panic disorder. *Psychiatry Res.* 2017;255:161-166.

Matochik JA, London ED, Yildiz BO, Ozata, M, Caglayan, S, DePaoli, AM, Wong, ML, & Licinio, J. Effect of leptin replacement on brain structure in genetically leptin-deficient adults. *J Clin Endocrinol Metab* 2005; 90: pp. 2851-2854.

Matthew J. McGuire and Makoto Ishii. Leptin dysfunction and Alzheimer's disease: evidence from cellular, animal, and human studies. *Cell Mol Neurobiol*. 2016 March; 36(2): 203–217.

McGregor, G., Harvey, J. 2017. Food for thought: Leptin regulation of hippocampal function and its role in Alzheimer's disease. *Neuropharmacology* doi: 10.1016/j.neuropharm.2017.09.038.

Meier U, Gressner AM (2004). Endocrine regulation of energy metabolism: review of pathobiochemical and clinical chemical aspects of leptin, ghrelin, adiponectin and resistin. *Clin Chem,* 50, 9, 1511-1525.

Miller GE, Freedland KE, Carney RM, Stetler CA, Banks WA. Pathways linking depression, adiposity, and inflammatory markers in healthy young adults. *Brain Behav Immun.* 2003 Aug;17(4):276-85. doi: 10.1016/s0889-1591(03)00057-6. PMID: 12831830.

Montague CT, Prins JB, Sanders L, Digby, JE, & O'Rahilly, S. Depot- and sex-specific differences in human leptin mRNA expression. Implications for the control of regional fat distribution. *Diabetes* 1997; 46: 342–347.

Monteleone P, Fabrazzo M, Tortorella A, Fuschino A, Maj M. Opposite modifications in circulating leptin and soluble leptin receptor across the eating disorder spectrum. *Mol Psychiatry.* 2002;7(6):641-6. doi: 10.1038/sj.mp.4001043. PMID: 12140788.

Monteleone P, Martiadis V, Colurico B, Maj M. Leptin secretion is related to chronicity and severity of illness in bulimia nervosa. *Psychosom Med* 2002; 64: 874– 9.

Morrison CD (2009). Leptin signaling in brain: A link between nutrition and cognition? *Biochim Biophys Acta* 1792:401-8.

Morton NM, Emilsson V, De Groot P, Pallett AL, Cawthorne MA (1999). Leptin signalling in pancreatic islets and clonal insulin-secreting cells. *Journal of Molecular Endocrinology*, 22, 173-184.

Münzberg H, Morrison CD (2015). Structure, production and signaling of leptin. *Metabolism* 64:13-23.

Nam S-Y, Kratzsch J, Wook Kim K, Rae Kim K, Lim S-K, Marcus C. Cerebrospinal Fluid and Plasma Concentrations of Leptin, NPY, andα-MSH in Obese Women and Their Relationship to Negative Energy Balance. *The Journal of Clinical Endocrinology & Metabolism.* 2001;86(10):4849-53.

Niswender KD, Gallis B, Blevins JE, Corson MA, Schwartz MW, Baskin DG. Immunocytochemical detection of phosphatidylinositol 3-kinase activation by insulin and leptin. *J. Histochem. Cytochem.* 2003; 51: 275–283.

Norrelund H, Gravholt CH, Englaro P, Blum WF, Rascher W, Chistiansen J, & Jorgensen, J. Increased levels but preserved diurnal variation of serum leptin in GH-deficient patients: lack of impact of different modes of GH administration. *European journal of endocrinology.* 1998;138(6):644-52.

Nyström F, Ekman B, Österlund M, Lindström, T, Öhman, KP, & Arnqvist, HJ. Serum leptin concentrations in a normal population and in GH deficiency: negative correlation with testosterone in men and effects of GH treatment. *Clin Endocrinol* 1997; 47: 191–198.

O'Rahilly S. 20 years of leptin: what we know and what the future holds. *Journal of Endocrinology.* 2014;223(1):E1-E3.

Oomura Y, Hori N, Shiraishi T, Fukunaga K, Takeda H, Tsuji M, Matsumiya, T, Ishibashi, M, Aou, S, Li, XL, Kohno, D, Uramura, K, Sougawa, H, Yada, T, Wayner, MJ, & Sasaki, K. Leptin facilitates learning and memory performance and enhances hippocampal CA1 long-term potentiation and CaMK II phosphorylation in rats. *Peptides.* 2006;27(11):2738-2749.

Ostlund RE Jr, Yang JW, Klein S, Gingerich R (1996). Relation between plasma leptin concentration and body fat, gender, diet, age, and metabolic covariates. *J Clin Endocrinol Metab* 81:3909-13.

Ozmen S, Şeker A, Demirci E. Ghrelin and leptin levels in children with anxiety disorders. *J Pediatr Endocrinol* Metab. 2019;32(10):1043-1047.

Panariello F, Polsinelli G, Borlido C, Monda M, De Luca V., The role of leptin in antipsychotic-induced weight gain: genetic and non-genetic factors, *J Obes.* 2012;2012:572848.

Paolisso G, Rizzo MR, Mone CM, Tagliamonte, MR, Gambardella, A, Riondino, M, Carella, C, Varricchio, M, & D'Onofrio, F. Plasma sex hormones are significantly associated with plasma leptin concentration in healthy subjects. *Clin Endocrinol* 1998; 48: 291–297.

Pelleymounter MA, Cullen MJ, Baker MB, Hecht R, Winters D, Boone T, & Collins, F. Effects of the obese gene product on body weight regulation in ob/ob mice. *Science.* 1995;269(5223):540-3.

Pelleymounter MA, Cullen MJ, Baker MB, Hecht R, Winters D, Boone T, & Collins, F. Effects of the obese gene product on body weight regulation in ob/ob mice. *Science.* 1995;269(5223):540-3.

Peña R, Marquina D, Serrano A, Elfakih, Y, Debaptista, E, Carrizo, E, Fernandez, V, Valery, L, Teneud, L, & Baptista, T. Frequency of abnormal correlation between leptin and the body mass index during first and second generation antipsychotic drug treatment, *Schizophr Res.* 2008;106(2-3):315-9.

Peterlin BL. The role of the adipocytokines adiponectin and leptin in migraine. *J Am Osteopath Assoc.* 2009;109(6):314-7.

Plum L, Belgardt BF, Bruning JC. Central insulin action in energy and glucose homeostasis. *J Clin Invest* 2006; 116: 1761-1766.

Quinton ND, Laird SM, Okon MA, Li, TC, Smith, RF, Blakemore, AI. Serum leptin levels during the menstrual cycle of healthy fertile women. *Br J Biomed Sci* 1999; 56: 16–19.

Randhawa BK, Farley BG, Boyd LA., Repetitive transcranial magnetic stimulation improves handwriting in Parkinson's disease, *Parkinsons Dis.* 2013;2013:751925.

Remesar X, Rafecas I, Femandez–Lopez JA, Alemany M. Is leptin an insülin counter-regulatory hormone?. *FEBS Leth* 1997; 402: 9-11.

Rentsch J, Chiesi M. Regulation of ob gene mRNA levels in cultured adipocytes. *FEBS Lett* 1996; 379: 55-9.

Roa J, Garcia-Galiano D, Castellano JM, Gaytan, F, Pinilla, L, & Tena-Sempere, M. Metabolic control of puberty onset: New players, new mechanisms. *Mol Cell Endocrinol* 2010;324:87–94.

Rosenbaum M, Murphy EM, Heymsfield SB, Matthews DE, Leibel RL. Low dose leptin administration reverses effects of sustained weight-reduction on energy expenditure and circulating concentrations of thyroid hormones. *The Journal of Clinical Endocrinology & Metabolism.* 2002;87(5):2391-4.

Rosenbaum M, Nicolson M, Hirsch J, Heymsfield SB, Gallagher D, Chu F, Leibel, RL. Effects of gender, body composition, and menopause on plasma concentrations of leptin. *The Journal of Clinical Endocrinology & Metabolism.* 1996;81(9):3424-7.

Rubin RT, Rhodes ME, Czambel RK. Sexual diergism of baseline plasma leptin and leptin suppression by arginine vasopressin in major depressives and matched controls. *Psychiatry Res*. 2002 Dec 30;113(3):255-68. doi: 10.1016/s0165-1781(02)00263-9. PMID: 12559482.

Santoro A, Mattace Raso G, Meli R. Drug targeting of leptin resistance. *Life Sciences*. 2015;140:64-74.

Scarpace PJ, Matheny M (1998). Leptin induction of UCP1 gene expression is dependent on sympathetic innervation. *Am J Physiol*, 275, 259-264.

Schapira AH., Recent developments in biomarkers in Parkinson disease, *Curr Opin Neurol*. 2013;26(4):395-400.

Schwartz MW, Peskind E, Raskind M, Boyko EJ, Porte D. Cerebrospinal fluid leptin levels: relationship to plasma levels and to adiposity in humans. *Nature medicine*. 1996;2(5):589.

Schwartz MW, Peskind E, Raskind M, Boyko EJ, Porte D. Cerebrospinal fluid leptin levels: relationship to plasma levels and to adiposity in humans. *Nature medicine*. 1996;2(5):589.

Schwartz MW, Seeley RJ (1997). Neuroendocrine responses to starvation and weight loss, *New Eng J Med*, 19, 1807-1811.

Schwartz MW, Seeley RJ, Woods SC. Wasting illness as a disorder of body weight regulation. *Proc. Nutr. Soc* 1997; 56: 785-191.

Schwartz MW, Woods SC, Porte D Jr, Seeley RJ, Baskin DG. Central nervous system control of food intake. *Nature* 2000; 404:661–671.

Seufert J. Leptin effects on pancreatic β-cell gene expression and function. Diabetes. 2004;53(suppl 1):S152-S8.

Shimabukuro M, Koyama K, Chen G, Wang, MY, Trieu, F, Lee, Y, Newgard, CB, & Unger, RH. Direct antidiabetic effect of leptin through triglyceride depletion of tissues. *Proc Natl Acad Sci USA* 1997; 94: 4637- 41.

Sinha MK, Ohannesian JP, Heiman ML, Kriauciunas A, Stephens TW, Magosin S, Marco, C, & Caro, JF. Nocturnal rise of leptin in lean, obese, and non-insulin-dependent diabetes mellitus subjects. *The Journal of clinical investigation*. 1996;97(5):1344-7.

Sinha MK, Opentanova I, Ohannesian JP, Kolaczynski JW, Heiman ML, Hale J (1996). Evidence of free and bound leptin in human circulation. *J Clin Invest* 98:1277–82.

Sinha MK. Human leptin: the hormone of adipose tissue. *Eur J Endocrinol* 1997; 136: 461-4.

Takayanagi Y, Cascella NG, Santora D, Gregory PE, Sawa A, Eaton WW. Relationships between serum leptin level and severity of positive symptoms in schizophrenia. *Neurosci Res*. 2013;77(1-2):97-101.

Tartaglia LA, Dembski M, Weng X, Deng N, Culpepper J, Devos R, ve ark. Identification and expression cloning of a leptin receptor, OB-R. *Cell* 1995; 83(7): 1263-71.

Tena-Sempere M. Roles of ghrelin and leptin in the control of reproductive function. *Neuroendocrinology* 2007; 86:229–41. 65.

Trayhurn P, Duncan JS, Rayner DV. Acute cold-induced suppression of ob (obese) gene expression in white adipose tissue of mice: mediation by the sympathetic system. *Biochem J* 1995; 311: 729- 33.

Ülker M, Kenangil G. The Relation of Circulating Levels of Leptin with Cognition in Patients with Alzheimer's Disease, *Arch Neuropsychiatry* 2018;55:211−214.

Van Aggel-Leijssen DPC, van Baak MA, Tenenbaum R, Campfield LA, Saris WHM (1999). Regulation of average 24h human plasma leptin level; the influence of exercise and physiological changes in energy balance. *Int J Obesity*, 23, 151–158.

Van Harmelen V, Reynisdottir S, Eriksson P, Thörne, A, Hoffstedt, J, Lönnqvist, F, & Arner, P. Leptin secretion from subcutaneous and visceral adipose tissue in women. *Diabetes* 1998; 47: 913–917.

Van Swieten MM, Pandit R, Adan RA, van der Plasse G (2014). The neuroanatomical function of leptin in the hypothalamus. *J Chem Neuroanat* 61-62:207-20.

Ve Hudetz JA, Gandhi SD, Iqbal Z, Patterso KM, Pagel PS. Elevated postoperative inflammatory biomarkers are associated with short- and medium-term cognitive dysfunction after coronary artery surgery. *J Anesth* 2011, 25:1–9.

Villareal D, Reams G, Freeman RH and Taraben A. Renal effects of leptin in normotensive, hypertensive, and obese rats. *The American Journal Physiology* 1998; 275: 2056-2060.

Warren MW, Hynan LS, Weiner MF., Lipids and adipokines as risk factors for Alzheimer's disease, *J Alzheimers Dis*. 2012;29(1):151-7.

Wolf G. Neuropeptides responding to leptin. *Nutr. Rev.* 1997; 55: 85-88.

Xu AW, Kaelin CB, Takeda K, Akira S, Schwartz MW, Barsh GS. PI3K integrates the action of insulin and leptin on hypothalamic neurons. *J. Clin. Invest.* 2005; 115: 951-958.

Yu Wh, Kimura M, Walczewska A, Karanth S, Mccann SM (1997). Role of leptin in hypothalamic-pituitary function. *P Natl Acad Sci USA*, 94, 1023-1028.

Zeki Al Hazzouri A, Haan MN, Whitmer RA, Yaffe K, Neuhaus J. Central obesity, leptin and cognitive decline: the Sacramento Area Latino Study on Aging. *Dement Geriatr Cogn Disord.* 2012;33(6):400-9.

Zemel MB. Agouti / melanocortin interactions with leptin pathways in obesity. *Nutr Rev* 1998; 56: 271–274.

Zeng J, Patterson BW, Klein S, Martin DR, Dagogo-Jack S, Kohrt WM, Miller SB, Landt M. 1997. Whole body leptin kinetics and renal metabolism in vivo. *Am J Physiol* 273, 1102–1106.

Zhang F, Chen Y, Heiman M, Dimarchi R (2005). Leptin: structure, function and biology. *Vitam Horm* 71:345-72.

Zhang F, Wang S, Signore AP, Chen J. Neuroprotective effects of leptin against ischemic injury induced by oxygenglucose deprivation and transient cerebral ischemia. *Stroke.* 2007;38(8):2329-36.

Zhang J, Deng Z, Liao J, Song, C, Liang, C, Xue, H, Wang, L, Zhang, K, & Yan, G. 2013. Leptin attenuates cerebral ischemia injury through the promotion of energy metabolism via the PI3K/Akt pathway. *J Cereb Blood Flow Metab.* 33(4):567-74.

Zhang Y, Chua S Jr (2017). Leptin function and regulation. *Compr Physiol* 8:351-369.

Zhang Y, Proenca R, Maffei M, Barone M, Leopold L, Friedman JM. 1994. Positional cloning of the mouse obese gene and its human homologue. *Nature* 372:425-32.

Zierath JR, Frevert EU, Ryder JW, Berggren PO, Kahn BB. 1998. Evidence against a direct effect of leptin on glucose transport in skeletal muscle and adipocytes. *Diabetes,* 47, 1-4.

Zlokovic BV, Jovanovic S, Miao W, Samara S, Verma S, Farrell CL. 2000. Differential regulation of leptin transport by the choroid plexus and blood-brain barrier and high affinity transport systems for entry into hypothalamus and across the bloodcerebrospinal fluid barrier. *Endocrinology* 141(4):1434 41.

Zupancic ML, Mahajan A. 2011. Leptin as a neuroactive agent. *Psychosom Med.* 73(5):407-14.

Chapter 2

The Role of Leptin as a Biochemical Marker in Health and Disease

Hadi Karimkhani[*]
Department of Biochemistry, School of Medicine, Istanbul Okan University, Istanbul, Türkey
Department of Stem Cell, Institute of Health Sciences, Eskisehir Osmangazi University, Eskisehir, Türkey

Abstract

Leptin is a hormone primarily produced by adipose tissue (fat cells) and is critical in regulating energy balance and metabolism (Martínez-Sánchez 2020; Abella et al. 2017). It functions as a satiety signal, which means it tells your brain when you've had enough to eat and helps regulate your appetite (Gioldasi et al. 2019). In addition, leptin affects the immune system, controls reproduction, and reduces inflammation (Francisco et al. 2018; Maurya et al. 2018).

In healthy individuals, leptin levels rise after eating, which helps to decrease appetite and increase energy expenditure. In people who are overweight or obese, however, leptin levels are often high, but their brains do not respond appropriately to the signal (Martínez-Sánchez 2020; Akeel Al-hussaniy, Hikmate Alburghaif, and Akeel Naji 2021). This condition is known as leptin resistance, and it can contribute to obesity, insulin resistance, and other metabolic disorders. Leptin deficiency is another condition that can lead to obesity and other health problems. People with congenital leptin deficiency have very low levels of leptin from birth, which leads to uncontrolled appetite and severe obesity. Treatment with synthetic leptin is effective in reducing appetite

---

[*] Corresponding Author's Email: drhadi.h@gmail.com.

In: Leptin and its Role in Health and Disease
Editor: Stephen E. Bradley
ISBN: 979-8-89113-274-0
© 2024 Nova Science Publishers, Inc.

and promoting weight loss in these individuals (Yupanqui-Lozno et al. 2019).

Leptin receptors are found on immune cells, and the hormone has been shown to influence the production and activity of inflammatory cytokines. Elevated leptin levels have been linked to rheumatoid arthritis and an increased risk of chronic inflammation and autoimmune diseases, including multiple sclerosis. Overall, leptin is a critical hormone that plays a central role in regulating energy balance, metabolism, and immune function. Research on the function of leptin in health and sickness is ongoing, and future findings may result in new treatments for various conditions (Abella et al. 2017; Cojocaru et al. 2013; Martínez-Sánchez 2020).

Keywords: leptin, leptin biochemical markers, leptin health, leptin disease, leptin metabolism, obesity

1. Introduction

1.1. Definition and Functions of Leptin Hormone

The hormone leptin is mainly produced by fat cells or adipose tissue. It is vital for controlling the body's metabolism and energy balance. As a satiety signal, leptin is the primary regulator of bodily energy levels, informing the brain (Pérez-Pérez et al. 2020).

When fat cells accumulate and expand, they release leptin into the bloodstream. After that, leptin reaches the brain, especially the hypothalamus, which controls hunger and energy expenditure. Leptin attaches to receptors in the brain and signals them to increase energy expenditure and decrease appetite (F. Zhang et al. 2005; Pérez-Pérez et al. 2020).

Structurally, leptin is a small protein hormone composed of 167 amino acids and the LEP gene, also known as the "OB gene". Human chromosome 7 is home to the LEP gene, which produces the hormone leptin. It is a member of the cytokine class, comprised of signalling molecules used in intercellular communication. After post-translational changes, leptin is produced as a preprohormone and becomes the active leptin molecule (Erichsen, Fadel, and Reagan 2022). The three-dimensional structure of leptin is made up of an alpha-helical bundle, a structural pattern that is common to many proteins. Four helices connected by short loops form the pile. Leptin's general structure provides stability and enables it to attach to target cells' leptin receptors (F. Zhang et al. 2005; Hammond et al. 2012).

On the other hand, abnormalities in metabolism and energy management may result from disturbances in leptin signaling. When the brain does not react to leptin's signals appropriately, it can lead to leptin resistance, a condition seen in obesity that increases hunger and decreases energy expenditure (Martínez-Sánchez 2020; Akeel Al-hussaniy, Hikmate Alburghaif, and Akeel Naji 2021).

In conclusion, leptin is a hormone that fat cells generate, essential for controlling hunger, metabolism, and energy balance. It affects inflammation and the immune system in addition to regulating energy. To fully grasp leptin's role in health and disease, one must know its fundamental description and functioning (Cojocaru et al. 2013; Babaei et al. 2011; Park and Ahima 2015; Francisco et al. 2018; Pérez-Pérez et al. 2020; Kiernan and MacIver 2021).

1.2. Overview of Biochemical Markers

When evaluating leptin's effects on health and illness, biochemical markers can be employed. For instance, researchers can investigate the connection between leptin and inflammation by measuring the levels of inflammatory markers like C-reactive protein (CRP) or cytokines. The association between leptin and metabolic diseases like diabetes or metabolic syndrome may also be investigated by analyzing metabolic indicators like insulin or glucose levels (Hribal, Fiorentino, and Sesti 2014).

Leptin is released into the bloodstream and travels to many tissues and organs, including the brain's hypothalamus, where it attaches to receptors to initiate action. When leptin binds to hypothalamic receptors, a series of signals are set off that lead to a reduction in hunger and an increase in energy expenditure (Park and Ahima 2015; Salazar et al. 2020).

Leptin stimulates the production of thyroid and growth hormones through a complex biochemical signaling pathway. Here's a brief overview of the mechanisms involved:

The JAK2-STAT3 signaling pathway is triggered by leptin attaching to its receptor in the hypothalamus, activating several transcription factors that control gene expression (Scabia et al. 2018).

1. The gene encoding the hypothalamic thyrotropin-releasing hormone (TRH) is one of the target genes controlled by leptin and STAT3 (Harris et al. 2001).

2. TRH releases thyroid-stimulating hormone (TSH) from the pituitary gland (Mullur, Liu, and Brent 2014).
3. TSH stimulates the thyroid gland to produce and release thyroid hormone (TH), which regulates metabolism and energy expenditure (Mullur, Liu, and Brent 2014).
4. Leptin also stimulates the release of growth hormone-releasing hormone (GHRH) from the hypothalamus (Luque et al. 2007).
5. GHRH, in turn, stimulates the release of growth hormone (GH) from the pituitary gland (Luque et al. 2007; Saleri et al. 2004).
6. Growth hormone (GH) stimulates the liver and other tissues to produce more insulin-like growth factor 1 (IGF-1), which promotes development and increases energy expenditure (Luque et al. 2007; Saleri et al. 2004).

By activating different signaling pathways and transcription factors that control gene expression, hormone synthesis, and release, leptin increases the biochemical processes that result in the generation of thyroid hormone and growth hormone. Increased metabolic rate and energy expenditure are the ultimate results of leptin's effects on thyroid hormone and growth hormone synthesis, which support energy balance and prevent obesity (Luque et al. 2007; Saleri et al. 2004).

Leptin changes how cells work through several signaling pathways, such as activating proteins like JAK2, IRS, MAPK, SOCS, and STAT (Allison and Myers 2014; Maymó et al. 2010). The following summarizes how leptin affects these proteins:

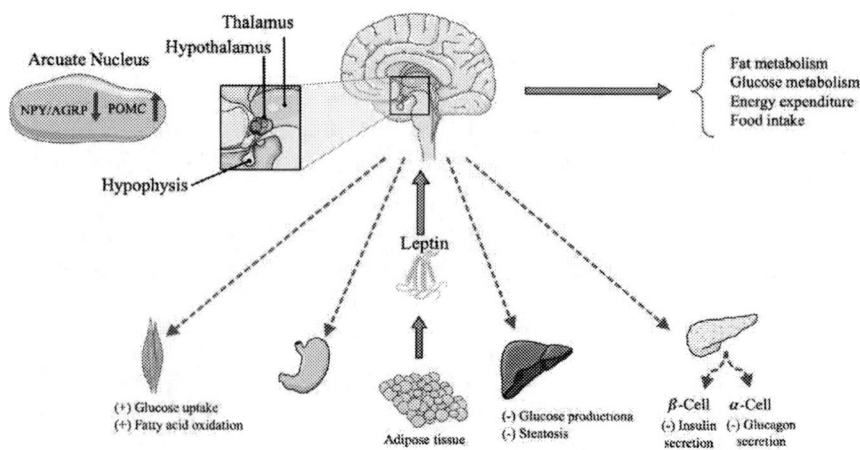

1.2.1. Signal Transducer and Activator of Transcription (STAT)

Leptin activates the STAT pathway by binding to its receptor on the cell surface. This binding triggers the activation of JAK2, which then phosphorylates and activates STAT proteins. Following activation, STAT proteins go to the nucleus, where they control the functioning of several genes involved in distinct biological functions, such as metabolic processes, inflammation, and immunity (Yi et al. 2017; Mullen and Gonzalez-Perez 2016; Zimmerman and Harris 2015; Landry et al. 2017).

1.2.2. Janus Kinase 2 (JAK2)

One protein that is essential to leptin signaling is called JAK2. JAK2 is triggered when leptin interacts with its receptor, phosphorylating particular tyrosine residues on the receptor and downstream signaling proteins, such as STAT. The activation of downstream signaling cascades due to this phosphorylation event ultimately affects cell function (Mullen and Gonzalez-Perez 2016; Landry et al. 2017; Jiang et al. 2021; Hadley, Cakir, and Cone 2020).

1.2.3. Mitogen-Activated Protein Kinase (MAPK)

Leptin can also activate the MAPK pathway, which is involved in cell proliferation, differentiation, and survival. Several proteins, including p38 MAPK, JNK (c-Jun N-terminal kinase), and ERK (extracellular signal-regulated kinase), can be phosphorylated as an effect of leptin's activation of MAPK. These phosphorylated proteins then regulate gene expression and cellular responses (Patraca et al. 2017; CHEN et al. 2014).

1.2.4. Insulin Receptor Substrate (IRS)

Leptin signaling can intersect with the insulin signaling pathway by activating IRS proteins. The activation of PI3K (phosphoinositide 3-kinase) and Akt is a downstream signaling pathway that phosphorylated IRS proteins mediate in response to leptin receptor activation. This signaling cascade is essential for regulating glucose metabolism and insulin sensitivity (Allison and Myers 2014; Gorgisen, Gulacar, and Ozes 2017).

1.2.5. Suppressor of Cytokine Signaling (SOCS)

Leptin signaling can induce the expression of SOCS proteins, which act as negative feedback regulators of the pathway. SOCS proteins inhibit leptin signaling by binding to the receptors or downstream signaling components, thereby dampening the activation of STAT and other signaling pathways (Howard and Flier 2006; Piessevaux et al. 2006).

Overall, leptin influences cell function by activating STAT, JAK2, MAPK, IRS, and the induction of SOCS proteins. The many effects of leptin on immunological response, metabolism, and other cellular functions are mediated by these signaling pathways.

A complicated molecular signaling route in the hypothalamus is how leptin interacts with receptors. Leptin binds to leptin receptors on the surface of particular hypothalamic neurons after being released by fat cells and reaching the hypothalamus (Scabia et al. 2018). When the leptin receptor binds leptin, it changes shape and activates the corresponding JAK2 as a type I cytokine receptor. Tyrosine residues on the intracellular signaling protein signal transducer and activator of STAT3 and the receptor itself get phosphorylated following JAK2 activation. When phosphorylated STAT3 separates from the receptor and forms homodimers or heterodimers, it travels to the nucleus and binds to certain promoter regions (Uchiyama et al. 2011; Thiagarajan et al. 2017). Cocaine- and amphetamine-regulated transcript (CART), proopiomelanocortin (POMC), and neuropeptide Y (NPY) are among the target genes controlled by leptin and STAT3. These genes stimulate hunger and enhance energy expenditure, respectively. (Belgardt, Okamura, and Brüning 2009; Scabia et al. 2018; Bouyer and Simerly 2013). Besides STAT3, leptin signaling triggers additional signaling pathways in the hypothalamus, including the PI3K and MAPK pathways. Gene expression alterations and the activation of more transcription factors may result from these pathways. Therefore, the leptin hormone controls our eating habits and energy balance through the brain (Atoum, Alzoughool, and Al-Hourani 2020; Kim and Kim 2021; Mullur, Liu, and Brent 2014).

For the most part, several signaling pathways and transcription factors are involved in the hypothalamus's intricate and strictly controlled process of leptin signaling. By suppressing hunger and increasing energy expenditure leptin ultimately achieves its goal of preventing obesity and maintaining energy balance in the body by attaching to its receptors in the brain. Nevertheless, while the brains have become less sensitive to the effects of leptin people who are overweight or obese may experience constant hunger and a decrease in energy expenditure. As well as other metabolic diseases, this may exacerbate weight gain. Since it stimulates energy expenditure and functions as a satiety signal, leptin is essential for controlling energy balance and metabolism. An additional factor in metabolic diseases, including obesity and insulin resistance is the dysregulation of leptin signaling (Tanida et al. 2015; Hadley, Cakir, and Cone 2020).

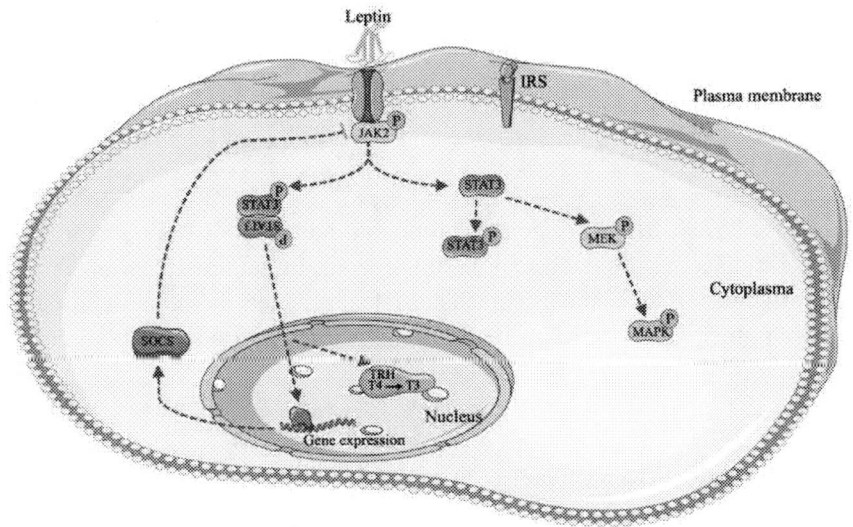

2. Effects of Function Leptin Hormone in the Body

2.1. Central Nervous System

Leptin's effects on ingestive behaviour, energy balance, and the reproductive system are mediated by neuronal networks in the central nervous system (Y. Zhang and Chua 2017).

2.2. Liver

The liver, the primary organ of systemic metabolism, is closely linked to leptin. It affects the liver both directly and indirectly. Understanding the hormonal and metabolic interactions between the liver and adipose tissue may identify novel treatment targets for certain chronic liver illnesses (Martínez-Uña et al. 2020).

2.3. Kidney

Chronic kidney disease (CKD) patients have hyperleptinemia linked to leptin regulation of kidney function. Elevated leptin may worsen renal function in individuals with CKD and raise cardiovascular risk (Korczynska et al. 2021).

2.4. Placenta

Maternal obesity affects placental function and fetal development, and changes in placental function may be involved in linking maternal obesity to long-term health risks in the infant. Maternal adipokines, including leptin, link maternal nutritional status and adipose tissue metabolism to placental function (Howell and Powell 2017; Maymó et al. 2012).

3. Leptin Resistance and the Association with Obesity

Leptin resistance is characterized by reduced sensitivity to the hormone leptin, despite high levels in the bloodstream. This condition is commonly associated with obesity (Mendoza-Herrera et al. 2021). Let's investigate the connection between obesity and leptin resistance:

3.1. Leptin's Role in Energy Regulation

Leptin functions as a satiety signal, advising the brain when to stop eating and how much energy to use. Therefore, it is essential for controlling energy balance in the body and metabolism. When we eat our body breaks down the food and releases nutrients like fatty acids and glucose into the bloodstream. This causes the pancreas to release insulin, which aids in delivering fatty acids and glucose into cells for cellular energy synthesis or storage. In response to increased nutrient availability, fat cells synthesize and secrete leptin into the bloodstream (Friedman 2019; Sutton, Myers, and Olson 2016). Various factors, including glucocorticoids, insulin, and inflammatory cytokines, regulate the process of leptin secretion. Insulin, inflammatory cytokines, and glucocorticoids are involved in regulating leptin synthesis. Glucocorticoids and insulin boost leptin production, while inflammatory cytokines like TNF-α and IL-6 can influence leptin synthesis based on the situation (Procaccini, Jirillo, and Matarese 2012; Akeel Al-hussaniy, Hikmate Alburghaif, and Akeel Naji 2021; Maurya et al. 2018; Dutta et al. 2012).

The primary role of leptin is to help maintain body weight and prevent excessive weight gain. By signaling the brain when energy stores are sufficient, leptin helps regulate food intake and energy balance. In individuals with normal leptin function, higher levels after a meal indicate satiety and reduced appetite (Pérez-Pérez et al. 2020).

3.2. Leptin Resistance and Obesity

In individuals with obesity, despite having high levels of leptin, the brain does not respond adequately to its signals. This reduced sensitivity to leptin is known as leptin resistance. Numerous variables, such as a high-fat diet and sedentary behavior, as well as genetic predisposition and chronic inflammation, might contribute to the development of leptin resistance (Park and Ahima 2015; Rehman, Akash, and Alina 2018; Hribal, Fiorentino, and Sesti 2014; Mendoza-Herrera et al. 2021).

3.3. Leptin Deficiency

Genetic changes that affect leptin production or function or its receptors may cause leptin deficiency. Additionally, certain medical conditions or treatments, such as lipodystrophy (a disorder characterized by the loss of fatty tissue) or damage to the hypothalamus (the brain region involved in appetite regulation), can also result in leptin deficiency. Obesity and low leptin levels are related in a complicated and varied way. While leptin replacement therapy has shown potential in some instances of obesity associated with a leptin deficit, it might not work for everyone. Obesity can also develop and worsen due to other factors, including nutrition, lifestyle, and genetic susceptibility (Yupanqui-Lozno et al. 2019; Martínez-Sánchez 2020; Beghini et al. 2021).

Congenital leptin deficiency, an uncommon genetic condition characterized by abnormalities in metabolism and extreme obesity, can result from leptin (LEP) gene mutations. Because of their extremely low or nonexistent leptin levels, these people have an insatiable desire and have gained weight since infancy. To sum up, The leptin hormone, a crucial modulator of energy balance and metabolism, is encoded by the LEP gene.

Mutations in the LEP gene can result in congenital leptin deficiency, an uncommon genetic condition marked by abnormalities in metabolism and extreme obesity (Dayal et al. 2018; Yupanqui-Lozno et al. 2019; Cagliyan et al. 2022; Torchen et al. 2022).

4. Leptin's Role in Inflammation

Inflammation and leptin are tightly related. Inflammatory processes within the body impact leptin levels, and leptin can reduce inflammation. The primary source of leptin, adipose tissue, secretes various pro-inflammatory chemicals. These compounds are involved in the chronic low-grade inflammation frequently seen in obese individuals. TNF-α and IL-6 are inflammatory cytokines that can increase leptin synthesis and release from adipose tissue. Thus, greater leptin levels may result from persistently raised levels of these pro-inflammatory cytokines in diseases like obesity (Martínez-Sánchez 2020; Kamareddine et al. 2021; Atoum, Alzoughool, and Al-Hourani 2020).

In summary, leptin affects the immunological system and inflammatory processes as well. Leptin affects immunological system responses and inflammation via several metabolic pathways, including the following:

1. T cells, macrophages, and monocytes are among the immune cells that leptin can directly stimulate. Certain immune cells have leptin receptors on their surface, and leptin binds to these receptors to initiate intracellular signaling pathways that result in the production of cytokines and chemokines. The immune cell recruitment and inflammatory response depend heavily on these chemicals (Souza-Almeida et al. 2021; Kiernan and MacIver 2021).
2. Leptin can regulate the function of immune cells by controlling the activity of genes responsible for immune cell activation, differentiation, and growth. Examples of genes linked to T cell growth and activation include interleukin-2 (IL-2) and its receptor, which leptin can increase in expression (Pérez-Pérez et al. 2020; Fernández-Riejos et al. 2010; Naylor and Petri 2016).
3. Leptin modulates the creation and elimination of inflammatory mediators, such as leukotrienes and histamine, which affect inflammatory cells' activity, such as mast cells and neutrophils (Milling 2019; Pertiwi et al. 2019).

4. Leptin can impact cortisol and corticotropin-releasing hormone (CRH), two additional hormones in the immunological response. The release of cortisol from the adrenal gland can be stimulated by leptin through the hypothalamus's stimulation of CRH production. Cortisol can depress the immune system and has strong anti-inflammatory properties (Fernández-Riejos et al. 2010; Gioldasi et al. 2019).

Fluoxetine is an antidepressant that can increase leptin sensitivity (Scabia et al. 2018). The biochemical routes, gene expression regulation, interaction with other hormones and mediators, and diverse signaling pathways are all part of the intricate biochemical mechanisms via which leptin affects inflammation and immune system functioning. Leptin's effects on immune cells and inflammatory mediators may affect the pathophysiology and recovery of inflammatory and autoimmune disorders. Additionally, leptin regulates inflammation and the immune system.

Pro-inflammatory cytokines and chemokines have been demonstrated to be stimulated by it, and this can lead to the development of chronic inflammation and associated illnesses (Cojocaru et al. 2013; Babaei et al. 2011; Park and Ahima 2015; Francisco et al. 2018; Pérez-Pérez et al. 2020; Kiernan and MacIver 2021).

Leptin is a hormone that has several mechanisms related to inflammation. Leptin can increase the production of specific cytokines, such as IL-6, that initiate an inflammatory response (Cojocaru et al. 2013). Leptin can also stimulate inflammation in T cells, macrophages, and other immune cells (Naylor and Petri 2016). Leptin has been shown to play a role in various diseases, including endometrial cancer (Madeddu et al. 2022; Elias and Purohit 2013), pulmonary inflammation (Maurya et al. 2018; Hammond et al. 2012), cardiac remodeling (Allison and Myers 2014; CHEN et al. 2014; Kamareddine et al. 2021), and joint inflammation (Cojocaru et al. 2013; Abella et al. 2017; Kamareddine et al. 2021). In endometrial cancer, leptin levels correlate with tumour size, disease stage, proinflammatory cytokines, and oxidative stress (Cojocaru et al. 2013). In pulmonary inflammation, leptin receptor signaling was found to sustain the metabolic fitness of alveolar macrophages and attenuate pulmonary inflammation (Guo et al. 2022). Dysregulation of the adipokines leptin and adiponectin in cardiac remodeling affected the heart's autophagic response and contributed to accelerating cardiac remodeling. In joint inflammation, leptin contributed to the pathogenesis of rheumatoid arthritis and its potential mechanisms. In nonalcoholic fatty liver disease, leptin-deficient mice showed liver structural injury, including steatosis, inflammation, and possible apoptosis linked to high Caspase 3 expression (Kamareddine et al. 2021).

Several biochemical markers have been associated with leptin levels and its dysregulation in disease states. These include glucose and insulin levels at fasting and indicators of insulin resistance such as TNF-α, IL-6, and C-reactive protein (CRP).

5. Leptin's Effect on Insulin Resistance

Insulin resistance refers to a condition in which cells become less responsive to the hormone insulin, leading to impaired glucose metabolism. The relationship between leptin and insulin resistance is complex. Here are the key points from the search results: Elevated leptin levels can interfere with insulin signaling, contributing to insulin resistance. Leptin can suppress insulin secretion by pancreatic beta cells and reduce insulin sensitivity in peripheral tissues such as skeletal muscle and liver (Hennige et al. 2006). Insulin resistance can alter leptin's effects on energy balance and appetite management by interfering with leptin signaling pathways. Research has demonstrated that compared to people without insulin resistance, obese people with insulin resistance have higher serum leptin levels (Erichsen, Fadel, and Reagan 2022). Visceral adipose tissue and body mass index (BMI), linked to insulin resistance, have been reported to correlate positively with leptin levels (Zarrati et al. 2019; Salazar et al. 2020; Park and Ahima 2015).

Leptin plays a complex role in diabetes development and management. Leptin levels are typically low or average in type 1 diabetes, brought on by the autoimmune destruction of pancreatic beta cells. However, leptin resistance frequently develops in type 2 diabetes, linked to insulin resistance. Although leptin levels are elevated, the brain cannot perceive leptin signals, leading to increased hunger and weight gain (Grasso 2022; Piessevaux et al. 2006; Akeel Al-hussaniy, Hikmate Alburghaif, and Akeel Naji 2021; Safai et al. 2015). Chronic inflammation may cause leptin resistance in type 2 diabetes, as it might obstruct leptin's capacity to penetrate the blood-brain barrier and control hunger. Leptin resistance can also contribute to insulin resistance by impairing insulin signaling in peripheral tissues such as muscle and the liver (F. Zhang et al. 2005; Y. Zhang and Chua 2017; Pérez-Pérez et al. 2020). However, leptin can also treat diabetes and other associated diseases. Treatment with leptin has been demonstrated to enhance glucose metabolism and insulin sensitivity in animal experiments. However, in humans, the use of leptin as a treatment for diabetes has been limited due to the development of leptin resistance and the lack of efficacy in clinical trials (Howard and Flier 2006; Rehman, Akash, and Alina 2018). In conclusion, leptin signaling modifications may contribute to the onset of insulin resistance and type 2 diabetes. Leptin has a complicated role in diabetes. Although leptin offers promise as a diabetic treatment, more investigation is required to comprehend its mechanisms and effectiveness in humans fully.

6. Leptin and Diseases

Leptin levels are closely related to an individual's overall health, and deviations from normal leptin levels can have implications for various aspects of health (Kiernan and MacIver 2021; Andò et al. 2019). Let's explore the relationship between leptin levels and overall health:

6.1. Obesity

Body fat mass has a significant impact on leptin levels. Leptin levels rise in obese people because they have more adipose tissue. Nonetheless, leptin resistance can arise in obesity and associated metabolic conditions such as type 2 diabetes and insulin resistance. Despite high circulating levels, Leptin resistance refers to reduced sensitivity to leptin's signals. This can disrupt appetite regulation, energy balance, and metabolic processes, contributing to the development and progression of metabolic health conditions (Kiernan and MacIver 2021).

6.2. Cardiovascular

There is a connection between leptin and cardiovascular health. An increased risk of cardiovascular diseases, including high blood pressure, atherosclerosis, and heart disease, has been associated with elevated leptin levels, primarily in the presence of obesity. Leptin may directly affect blood vessels by encouraging oxidative stress, vasoconstriction, and inflammation—all of which may play a role in the emergence of cardiovascular problems (De Rosa et al. 2009; Demir et al. 2018).

High levels of leptin have been linked to an increased risk of atherosclerosis, heart disease, and hypertension, among other cardiovascular disorders, especially when obesity is present. Leptin controls cardiovascular health through several essential pathways by directly influencing blood vessels. Leptin can stimulate vasoconstriction, oxidative stress, and inflammation, all of which can aid in the onset and advancement of cardiovascular problems (Kamareddine et al. 2021; Korczynska et al. 2021).

One inflammatory biomarker frequently used to predict the risk of cardiovascular disease is C-reactive protein or CRP. It has been demonstrated that leptin causes adipose tissue and liver cells to produce more CRP (Singh et al. 2007; Hribal, Fiorentino, and Sesti 2014). Furthermore, circulating inflammatory cytokines like IL-6, which stimulate the manufacture of CRP, are primarily sourced from adipocytes. The liver and vasculature can directly produce more CRP when leptin is present. According to molecular research, leptin can stimulate endothelium and hepatocyte cells to produce CRP in vitro. Administration of leptin in vivo has the potential to alter plasma CRP levels. Two investigations have shown that CRP binds directly to leptin in extracellular environments, reducing biological effects (Hribal, Fiorentino, and Sesti 2014). The physiological and molecular processes underlying the complicated relationship between leptin and CRP remain unclear (Farooqi and O'Rahilly 2007; Viikari et al. 2007; Chiu et al. 2012; Hribal, Fiorentino, and Sesti 2014; Singh et al. 2007).

Leptin controls the cytokine IL-6, which is involved in inflammation and the immune system. When leptin is present, immune cells such as monocytes, macrophages, and T cells can release more IL-6 (Tazawa et al. 2019; Torpy, Bornstein, and Chrousos 1998; Yang et al. 2013). Elevated serum levels of proinflammatory cytokines, including IL-6 and leptin, may indicate a chronic inflammatory state in schizophrenia patients, according to a preliminary investigation (Neelamekam, Nurjono, and Lee 2014). The hypothalamic-pituitary-adrenal axis is stimulated by IL-6 and inhibited by leptin (Torpy, Bornstein, and Chrousos 1998).

Firstly, leptin has been shown to induce inflammation within the blood vessel walls. This inflammatory response can lead to the recruitment of immune cells and the release of proinflammatory molecules, triggering a cascade of events that promote atherosclerotic plaque formation. These plaques, composed of cholesterol and other substances, can obstruct blood flow and increase the risk of developing conditions such as coronary artery disease (Korczynska et al. 2021; De Rosa et al. 2009).

Moreover, leptin can enhance oxidative stress within the vasculature. Reactive oxygen species (ROS) generation and the body's capacity to neutralize them are out of balance, which leads to oxidative stress. Excessive ROS production can damage the endothelial lining of blood vessels, impairing their function and promoting the development of atherosclerosis (Korczynska et al. 2021).

Additionally, leptin has vasoconstrictive effects, meaning it can cause the narrowing of blood vessels. This constriction can lead to increased peripheral resistance and elevated blood pressure, contributing to the development of hypertension. Furthermore, the narrowing of blood vessels can limit the delivery of oxygen and nutrients to vital organs, including the heart, further exacerbating the risk of cardiovascular complications. Leptin has been implicated in cardiovascular health. Elevated levels of leptin, especially in the context of obesity, have been associated with an increased risk of cardiovascular diseases such as hypertension, atherosclerosis, and heart disease. Leptin can directly affect blood vessels, promoting inflammation, oxidative stress, and vasoconstriction, contributing to cardiovascular complications (Kamareddine et al. 2021; Korczynska et al. 2021).

6.3. Reproductive

Leptin plays a crucial role in reproductive health, particularly in women. It is involved in regulating menstrual cycles and fertility, and both low and high levels of leptin can significantly impact reproductive function (Nillni 2010; Elias and Purohit 2013).

Low levels of leptin, often observed in conditions such as hypothalamic amenorrhea, can disrupt the normal functioning of the reproductive system. Low energy availability is a defining feature of hypothalamic amenorrhea, typically due to excessive exercise, severe caloric restriction, or ongoing stress. In this condition, the low levels of leptin signal to the hypothalamus that the body is in an energy-deficient state, suppressing reproductive hormones. As a result, menstrual irregularities, such as amenorrhea (absence of menstruation) or oligomenorrhea (infrequent or irregular menstruation), can occur. Furthermore, disrupting the hormonal balance can lead to anovulation (lack of ovulation) and infertility (Park and Ahima 2015; Elias and Purohit 2013; Martínez-Sánchez 2020; Fernanda and Fernandes 2014).

On the other hand, elevated leptin levels, as seen in conditions like polycystic ovary syndrome (PCOS), can also adversely affect reproductive health. PCOS is a common endocrine disorder characterized by insulin resistance, hyperandrogenism (elevated levels of male hormones), and ovarian dysfunction. In PCOS, the increased levels of leptin contribute to the disruption of ovulation, leading to irregular or absent menstrual cycles. The elevated leptin levels can further exacerbate insulin resistance, creating a vicious cycle that contributes to the pathogenesis of PCOS. The combination of insulin resistance and high leptin can disrupt the average hormonal balance, impair follicular development, and increase the risk of infertility (Wauters, Considine, and Van Gaal 2000; Akeel Al-hussaniy, Hikmate Alburghaif, and Akeel Naji 2021).

It is important to note that the precise mechanisms through which leptin affects reproductive health are complex and not yet fully understood. Leptin interacts with several other hormones and signaling pathways, such as insulin, follicle-stimulating hormone (FSH), luteinizing hormone (LH), gonadotropin-releasing hormone (GnRH), and luteinizing hormone (H), that are involved in reproductive function. The intricate interplay between these factors contributes to regulating menstrual cycles, ovulation, and fertility (Atoum, Alzoughool, and Al-Hourani 2020; Nillni 2010).

Understanding the role of leptin in reproductive health is essential for diagnosing and managing conditions such as hypothalamic amenorrhea and PCOS. Targeted interventions to restore leptin levels within the appropriate range, address underlying hormonal imbalances, and promote overall metabolic health may help restore normal reproductive function in individuals affected by these conditions (Wauters, Considine, and Van Gaal 2000; Akeel Al-hussaniy, Hikmate Alburghaif, and Akeel Naji 2021; Yupanqui-Lozno et al. 2019).

6.4. Bone Disorder

Leptin has been recognized as a regulator of bone metabolism. It plays a crucial role in maintaining bone health, and both low and high levels of leptin can significantly impact bone density and the risk of osteoporosis (Friedman 2019; Tsuchiya and Fujio 2022).

Low leptin levels, as observed in conditions such as anorexia nervosa or low body weight, can be associated with decreased bone mineral density and an increased risk of osteoporosis. Anorexia nervosa is an eating disorder characterized by severe caloric restriction and weight loss, leading to chronic energy deficiency. In individuals with anorexia nervosa or meager body weight, leptin levels are typically reduced. This decrease in leptin signaling can disrupt the average balance between bone formation and resorption, favouring bone loss. Leptin deficiency can impair osteoblast function, the cells responsible for bone formation. Additionally, it can enhance bone resorption, the process by which old bone tissue is broken down and replaced with new bone. The net effect of these disruptions is a reduction in bone mineral density and an increased risk of osteoporosis, a condition characterized by weak and brittle bones (Martínez-Sánchez 2020; Hebebrand et al. 2022).

Conversely, high levels of leptin, typically observed in conditions such as obesity, can also have implications for bone health. While obesity is generally associated with higher bone mineral density, the relationship between leptin and bone health in the context of obesity is complex. In obesity, excessive adipose tissue accumulation leads to elevated leptin levels. However, despite higher leptin levels, obese individuals may still experience adverse effects on bone health. Chronic inflammation and metabolic disturbances associated with obesity can impair bone quality and increase the risk of fractures (Shapses, Pop, and Wang 2017; Upadhyay, Farr, and Mantzoros 2015).

The precise mechanisms through which leptin influences bone metabolism are multifaceted and involve interactions with various signaling pathways and cells within the bone microenvironment. Leptin receptors are expressed on osteoblasts, osteoclasts (cells responsible for bone resorption), and bone marrow cells, indicating that leptin can directly influence bone cell function. Leptin also interacts with other hormones and factors involved in bone regulation, such as estrogen and insulin-like growth factor 1 (IGF-1). These interactions further contribute to the complex interplay between leptin and bone metabolism (Shapses, Pop, and Wang 2017; Atoum, Alzoughool, and Al-Hourani 2020; Hamrick et al. 2015).

Understanding the role of leptin in bone health is essential for developing strategies to prevent and treat conditions such as osteoporosis. Targeted interventions to restore leptin levels within the appropriate range, promote a healthy body weight, and address underlying metabolic imbalances may help improve bone health and reduce the risk of fractures (Shapses, Pop, and Wang 2017).

1. *Leptin and Hormonal Interactions:* Leptin interacts with other hormones involved in bone metabolism, such as estrogen and insulin-like growth factor 1 (IGF-1). Estrogen, for example, enhances adipose tissue's production and secretion of leptin. Leptin can modulate estrogen production and signaling pathways in bone cells. Estrogen

deficiency, naturally occurring during menopause or in conditions like primary ovarian insufficiency, can decrease leptin levels and contribute to bone loss. Similarly, leptin can affect IGF-1, a hormone that encourages bone growth. Leptin can stimulate the production of IGF-1, which further supports bone formation and mineralization (Hamrick et al. 2015; Atoum, Alzoughool, and Al-Hourani 2020; Binai et al. 2013).

2. *Leptin and the Bone Microenvironment:* Leptin acts directly on bone cells and affects the microenvironment. It has been found to modulate the production and secretion of various factors within the bone, including cytokines and growth factors. These factors play crucial roles in bone remodeling and can influence the activity of osteoblasts and osteoclasts. By regulating the bone microenvironment, leptin helps maintain a healthy balance between bone formation and resorption (Shapses, Pop, and Wang 2017; Upadhyay, Farr, and Mantzoros 2015).

3. *Leptin and Mechanical Loading:* Mechanical loading, such as weight-bearing exercise, is essential for maintaining bone health. Leptin has been shown to respond to mechanical loading, and its levels can increase during exercise. This suggests that leptin may mediate between automatic loading and bone metabolism. By sensing mechanical forces, leptin may help coordinate bone remodeling processes and adapt bone structure in response to changes in mechanical demands (Grasso 2022).

4. *Leptin's Therapeutic Potential:* Due to its involvement in bone metabolism, leptin has been investigated as a possible treatment target for diseases like osteoporosis that are linked to bone loss. Research has examined the impact of leptin receptor agonists or supplements on bone strength and density. More investigation is necessary to completely comprehend the possible advantages and restrictions of focusing on leptin for bone health therapies (Francisco et al. 2018; Sutton, Myers, and Olson 2016).

6.5. Autoimmune

Leptin has immunomodulatory effects and is involved in immune system regulation. It can influence both innate and adaptive immune responses. Dysregulation of leptin levels, such as in obesity or autoimmune diseases, can contribute to altered immune function and inflammation. Abnormal leptin levels have been associated with increased susceptibility to infections, impaired wound healing, and autoimmune disorders (Procaccini, Jirillo, and Matarese 2012; Babaei et al. 2011; Binai et al. 2013). It's important to note that while leptin levels can provide insights into overall health, they should be considered in conjunction with other clinical and laboratory parameters to comprehensively assess an individual's health status.

Leptin has been implicated in the pathogenesis of certain autoimmune diseases. Autoimmune diseases involve an abnormal immune response where the immune system mistakenly attacks healthy tissues. Leptin and its receptors are expressed in various immune cells, and leptin can modulate immune function. Abnormal leptin levels and signaling have been observed in autoimmune diseases such as rheumatoid arthritis, systemic lupus erythematosus, and multiple sclerosis. Dysregulation of leptin levels and signaling in these conditions may contribute to altered immune responses and disease progression (Kiernan and MacIver 2021; Babaei et al. 2011).

6.6. Cancer

Leptin, an obesity-associated adipokine, can promote cancer by enhancing inflammation. Chronic inflammation has been linked to the development of several types of cancer, and leptin can increase the production of pro-inflammatory cytokines such as IL-6 and TNF-a. These cytokines can promote inflammation and contribute to the development of cancer (de Candia et al. 2021; Dutta et al. 2012; Garofalo and Surmacz 2006; Lin and Hsiao 2021).

Certain forms of cancer have been linked to leptin's genesis and progression. Recent research has demonstrated the expression of leptin and leptin receptors in specific cell types, especially in tumour microenvironments and malignancies, and has delineated the function of this signaling pathway in the advancement of cancer (Lin and Hsiao 2021). Strong epidemiological evidence suggests that being very obese affects the prognosis, course, and chance of developing several cancers, including breast cancer (Andò et al. 2019). The precise processes behind the intricate link between leptin and cancer remain unclear. But according to specific research, leptin may, via various mechanisms, encourage the growth and spread of tumours (Atoum, Alzoughool, and Al-Hourani 2020; Andò et al. 2019; Lin and Hsiao 2021). Leptin can potentially exacerbate cancer by inducing angiogenesis, developing new blood vessels that provide oxygen and nutrition to tumours.

Vascular endothelial growth factor (VEGF), a protein that encourages angiogenesis, can be produced in response to leptin. This may accelerate the development of blood vessels in tumours, enabling the growth and spread of the tumour (Lin and Hsiao 2021).

Multiple research has expounded on leptin's significance in cancer development. Studies have indicated that dysregulation of the leptin/leptin receptor may play a part in the emergence of a wide range of cancers, including endometrial, breast, thyroid, and gastrointestinal malignancies. This involvement is primarily through the JAK/STAT pathway, which regulates the expression of antiapoptotic proteins (e.g., XIAP), systemic inflammation (e.g., TNF-α, IL6), angiogenic factors (VEGF), and hypoxia-inducible factor-1a (HIF-1a) (Dutta et al. 2012). Tumour cell survival can be enhanced by leptin through inducing differentiation of LEPR-positive cancer stem cells. These data demonstrate the therapeutic potential of leptin and leptin signaling for forming breast tumours (Allison and Myers 2014).

Conclusion

Leptin plays a significant role as a biochemical marker in health and disease. This hormone is crucial for controlling energy balance and metabolism (Abella et al. 2017; Cojocaru et al. 2013; Martínez-Sánchez 2020). Leptin functions as a satiety signal, informing the brain when enough food has been consumed and regulating appetite. Additionally, it affects the immune system, reproductive control, and inflammation reduction (F. Zhang et al. 2005; Pérez-Pérez et al. 2020).

In healthy individuals, leptin levels increase after eating, leading to decreased appetite and increased energy expenditure. However, in overweight or obese individuals, leptin levels are often high, but the brain does not respond appropriately to the signal. This condition, leptin resistance, can contribute to obesity, insulin resistance, and other metabolic disorders (Martínez-Sánchez 2020; Akeel Al-hussaniy, Hikmate Alburghaif, and Akeel Naji 2021; Yupanqui-Lozno et al. 2019). Leptin deficiency is another condition that can lead to obesity and other health problems. Individuals with congenital leptin deficiency have deficient levels from birth, resulting in uncontrolled appetite and severe obesity. Treatment with synthetic leptin has proven effective in reducing hunger and promoting weight loss in these individuals (Dayal et al. 2018; Yupanqui-Lozno et al. 2019; Cagliyan et al. 2022; Torchen et al. 2022).

Leptin receptors are found on immune cells, and the hormone has been shown to influence the production and activity of inflammatory cytokines. Elevated leptin levels have been linked to rheumatoid arthritis and an increased risk of chronic inflammation and autoimmune diseases, including multiple sclerosis. Leptin is a critical hormone that plays a central role in regulating energy balance, metabolism, and immune function. Ongoing research on the role of leptin in health and disease may lead to new treatments for various conditions (Procaccini, Jirillo, and Matarese 2012; Babaei et al. 2011; Binai et al. 2013).

This study represents an essential step in understanding the role of leptin as a biochemical marker in health and disease. Measuring leptin levels and investigating other biochemical markers associated with leptin can help diagnose and treat obesity, metabolic syndrome, inflammation, and other diseases. Future research may contribute to a better understanding of leptin and its associated mechanisms, leading to more effective management of health issues.

References

Abella, Vanessa, Morena Scotece, Javier Conde, Jesús Pino, Miguel Angel Gonzalez-Gay, Juan J. Gómez-Reino, Antonio Mera, Francisca Lago, Rodolfo Gómez, and Oreste Gualillo. 2017. "Leptin in the Interplay of Inflammation, Metabolism and Immune System Disorders." *Nature Reviews Rheumatology* 13 (2): 100–109. https://doi.org/10.1038/nrrheum.2016.209.

Akeel Al-hussaniy, Hany, Ali Hikmate Alburghaif, and Meena Akeel Naji. 2021. "Leptin Hormone and Its Effectiveness in Reproduction, Metabolism, Immunity, Diabetes, Hopes and Ambitions." *Journal of Medicine and Life* 14 (5): 600–605. https://doi.org/10.25122/jml-2021-0153.

Allison, Margaret B., and Martin G. Myers. 2014. "20 YEARS OF LEPTIN: Connecting Leptin Signaling to Biological Function." *Journal of Endocrinology* 223 (1): T25–35. https://doi.org/10.1530/JOE-14-0404.

Andò, Sebastiano, Luca Gelsomino, Salvatore Panza, Cinzia Giordano, Daniela Bonofiglio, Ines Barone, and Stefania Catalano. 2019. "Obesity, Leptin and Breast Cancer: Epidemiological Evidence and Proposed Mechanisms." *Cancers* 11 (1): 62. https://doi.org/10.3390/cancers11010062.

Atoum, Manar Fayiz, Foad Alzoughool, and Huda Al-Hourani. 2020. "Linkage Between Obesity Leptin and Breast Cancer." *Breast Cancer: Basic and Clinical Research* 14 (January): 117822341989845. https://doi.org/10.1177/1178223419898458.

Babaei, Arash, Sayyed Hamid Zarkesh-Esfahani, Ehsan Bahrami, and Richard Ross. 2011. "Restricted Leptin Antagonism as a Therapeutic Approach to Treatment of

Autoimmune Diseases." *HORMONES* 10 (1): 16–26. https://doi.org/10.14310/horm.2002.1289.

Beghini, Marianna, Stephanie Brandt, Ingrid Körber, Katja Kohlsdorf, Heike Vollbach, Belinda Lennerz, Christian Denzer, Shlomit Shalitin, Ferruccio Santini, Werner F. Blum, Julia von Schnurbein, and Martin Wabitsch. 2021. "Serum IGF1 and Linear Growth in Children with Congenital Leptin Deficiency before and after Leptin Substitution." *International Journal of Obesity 2021 45:7* 45 (7): 1448–56. https://doi.org/10.1038/s41366-021-00809-2.

Belgardt, Bengt F., Tomoo Okamura, and Jens C. Brüning. 2009. "Hormone and Glucose Signalling in POMC and AgRP Neurons." *The Journal of Physiology* 587 (22): 5305–14. https://doi.org/10.1113/jphysiol.2009.179192.

Binai, Nadine A., Gert Carra, Johannes Löwer, Roswitha Löwer, and Silja Wessler. 2013. "Differential Gene Expression in ERα-Positive and ERα-Negative Breast Cancer Cells upon Leptin Stimulation." *Endocrine* 44 (2): 496–503. https://doi.org/10.1007/s12020-013-9897-y.

Bouyer, Karine, and Richard B. Simerly. 2013. "Neonatal Leptin Exposure Specifies Innervation of Presympathetic Hypothalamic Neurons and Improves the Metabolic Status of Leptin-Deficient Mice." *The Journal of Neuroscience* 33 (2): 840–51. https://doi.org/10.1523/JNEUROSCI.3215-12.2013.

Cagliyan, Erkan, Samican Ozmen, Hikmet T. Timur, Mehmet E. Ozgozen, and Gokcen G. Semiz. 2022. "Morbidly Obese Pregnant Woman with Congenital Leptin Deficiency: Follow-up and Obstetric Outcome." *Journal of Obstetrics and Gynaecology Research* 48 (11): 2964–67. https://doi.org/10.1111/jog.15379.

Candia, Paola de, Francesco Prattichizzo, Silvia Garavelli, Carlo Alviggi, Antonio La Cava, and Giuseppe Matarese. 2021. "The Pleiotropic Roles of Leptin in Metabolism, Immunity, and Cancer." *Journal of Experimental Medicine* 218 (5). https://doi.org/10.1084/jem.20191593.

Chen, Jingfu, Hailiang Mo, Runmin Guo, Qiong You, Ruina Huang, and Keng Wu. 2014. "Inhibition of the Leptin-Induced Activation of the P38 MAPK Pathway Contributes to the Protective Effects of Naringin against High Glucose-Induced Injury in H9c2 Cardiac Cells." *International Journal of Molecular Medicine* 33 (3): 605–12. https://doi.org/10.3892/ijmm.2014.1614.

Chiu, Feng-Hsiang, Chung Hsun Chuang, Wen-Cheng Li, Yi-Ming Weng, Wen-Chih Fann, Hsiang-Yun Lo, Cheng Sun, and Shih-Hao Wang. 2012. "The Association of Leptin and C-Reactive Protein with the Cardiovascular Risk Factors and Metabolic Syndrome Score in Taiwanese Adults." *Cardiovascular Diabetology* 11 (1): 40. https://doi.org/10.1186/1475-2840-11-40.

Cojocaru, Manole, Inimioara Mihaela Cojocaru, Isabela Siloşi, and Suzana Rogoz. 2013. "Role of Leptin in Autoimmune Diseases." *Maedica* 8 (1): 68–74. /pmc/articles/PMC3749767/.

Dayal, Devi, Keerthivasan Seetharaman, Inusha Panigrahi, Balasubramaniyan Muthuvel, and Ashish Agarwal. 2018. "Severe Early Onset Obesity Due to a Novel Missense Mutation in Exon 3 of the Leptin Gene in an Infant from Northwest India." *Journal of Clinical Research in Pediatric Endocrinology* 10 (3): 274–78. https://doi.org/10.4274/jcrpe.5501.

Demir, S., G. Erten, B. Artım-Esen, Y. Şahinkaya, Ö Pehlivan, N. Alpay-Kanıtez, G. Deniz, and M. Inanç. 2018. "Increased Serum Leptin Levels Are Associated with Metabolic Syndrome and Carotid Intima Media Thickness in Premenopausal Systemic Lupus Erythematosus Patients without Clinical Atherosclerotic Vascular Events." *Lupus* 27 (9): 1509–16. https://doi.org/10.1177/0961203318782424.

Dutta, Deep, Sujoy Ghosh, Kaushik Pandit, Pradip Mukhopadhyay, and Subhankar Chowdhury. 2012. "Leptin and Cancer: Pathogenesis and Modulation." *Indian Journal of Endocrinology and Metabolism* 16 (9): 596. https://doi.org/10.4103/2230-8210.105577.

Elias, Carol F., and Darshana Purohit. 2013. "Leptin Signaling and Circuits in Puberty and Fertility." *Cellular and Molecular Life Sciences* 70 (5): 841–62. https://doi.org/10.1007/s00018-012-1095-1.

Erichsen, Jennifer M., Jim R. Fadel, and Lawrence P. Reagan. 2022. "Peripheral versus Central Insulin and Leptin Resistance: Role in Metabolic Disorders, Cognition, and Neuropsychiatric Diseases." *Neuropharmacology* 203 (February): 108877. https://doi.org/10.1016/j.neuropharm.2021.108877.

Farooqi, I. Sadaf, and Stephen O'Rahilly. 2007. "Is Leptin an Important Physiological Regulator of CRP?" *Nature Medicine* 13 (1): 16–17. https://doi.org/10.1038/nm0107-16.

Fernanda, Maria, and Andrade Fernandes. 2014. "Leptin Modulation of Locomotor and Emotional Behaviors: The Role of STAT3 Signaling in Dopamine Neurons."

Fernández-Riejos, Patricia, Souad Najib, Jose Santos-Alvarez, Consuelo Martín-Romero, Antonio Pérez-Pérez, Carmen González-Yanes, and Víctor Sánchez-Margalet. 2010. "Role of Leptin in the Activation of Immune Cells." *Mediators of Inflammation* 2010: 1–8. https://doi.org/10.1155/2010/568343.

Francisco, Vera, Jesús Pino, Victor Campos-Cabaleiro, Clara Ruiz-Fernández, Antonio Mera, Miguel A Gonzalez-Gay, Rodolfo Gómez, and Oreste Gualillo. 2018. "Obesity, Fat Mass and Immune System: Role for Leptin." *Frontiers in Physiology* 9 (June). https://doi.org/10.3389/fphys.2018.00640.

Friedman, Jeffrey M. 2019. "Leptin and the Endocrine Control of Energy Balance." *Nature Metabolism* 1 (8): 754–64. https://doi.org/10.1038/s42255-019-0095-y.

Garofalo, Cecilia, and Eva Surmacz. 2006. "Leptin and Cancer." *Journal of Cellular Physiology* 207 (1): 12–22. https://doi.org/10.1002/jcp.20472.

Gioldasi, Sofia, Alexia Karvela, Andrea Paola Rojas-Gil, Maria Rodi, Anne-Lise de Lastic, Iason Thomas, Bessie E. Spiliotis, and Athanasia Mouzaki. 2019. "Metabolic Association between Leptin and the Corticotropin Releasing Hormone." *Endocrine, Metabolic & Immune Disorders - Drug Targets* 19 (4): 458–66. https://doi.org/10.2174/1871530319666190206165626.

Gorgisen, G., I. M. Gulacar, and O. N. Ozes. 2017. "The Role of Insulin Receptor Substrate (IRS) Proteins in Oncogenic Transformation." *Cellular and Molecular Biology* 63 (1): 1. https://doi.org/10.14715/cmb/2017.63.1.1.

Grasso, Patricia. 2022. "Harnessing the Power of Leptin: The Biochemical Link Connecting Obesity, Diabetes, and Cognitive Decline." *Frontiers in Aging Neuroscience* 14 (April). https://doi.org/10.3389/fnagi.2022.861350.

Guo, Ziyi, Haoqi Yang, Jing-Ren Zhang, Wenwen Zeng, and Xiaoyu Hu. 2022. "Leptin Receptor Signaling Sustains Metabolic Fitness of Alveolar Macrophages to Attenuate Pulmonary Inflammation." *Science Advances* 8 (28): 3064. https://doi.org/10.1126/sciadv.abo3064.

Hadley, Colleen, Isin Cakir, and Roger D Cone. 2020. "SAT-604 The Role of the Focal Adhesion Kinase Family in Leptin Receptor Signaling." *Journal of the Endocrine Society* 4 (Supplement_1). https://doi.org/10.1210/jendso/bvaa046.666.

Hammond, John A., Chris Hauton, Kimberley A. Bennett, and Ailsa J. Hall. 2012. "Phocid Seal Leptin: Tertiary Structure and Hydrophobic Receptor Binding Site Preservation during Distinct Leptin Gene Evolution." Edited by Nikolas Nikolaidis. *PLoS ONE* 7 (4): e35395. https://doi.org/10.1371/journal.pone.0035395.

Hamrick, M. W., A. Dukes, P. Arounleut, C. Davis, S. Periyasamy-Thandavan, S. Mork, S. Herberg, M. H. Johnson, C. M. Isales, W. D. Hill, L. Otvos, Jr., and E. J. Belin de Chantemèle. 2015. "The Adipokine Leptin Mediates Muscle- and Liver-Derived IGF-1 in Aged Mice." *Experimental Gerontology* 70 (October): 92–96. https://doi.org/10.1016/j.exger.2015.07.014.

Harris, Mark, Carl Aschkenasi, Carol F. Elias, Annie Chandrankunnel, Eduardo A. Nillni, Christian Bjørbæk, Joel K. Elmquist, Jeffrey S. Flier, and Anthony N. Hollenberg. 2001. "Transcriptional Regulation of the Thyrotropin-Releasing Hormone Gene by Leptin and Melanocortin Signaling." *Journal of Clinical Investigation* 107 (1): 111–20. https://doi.org/10.1172/JCI10741.

Hebebrand, Johannes, Stefanie Zorn, Jochen Antel, Julia von Schnurbein, Martin Wabitsch, and Gertraud Gradl-Dietsch. 2022. "First Account of Psychological Changes Perceived by a Female with Congenital Leptin Deficiency upon Treatment with Metreleptin." *Obesity Facts* 15 (5): 730–35. https://doi.org/10.1159/000526169.

Hennige, Anita M., Norbert Stefan, Katja Kapp, Rainer Lehmann, Cora Weigert, Alexander Beck, Klaus Moeschel, Joanne Mushack, Erwin Schleicher, Hans-Ulrich Häring. 2006. "Leptin Down-regulates Insulin Action through Phosphorylation of Serine-318 in Insulin Receptor Substrate 1." *The FASEB Journal* 20 (8): 1206–8. https://doi.org/10.1096/fj.05-4635fje.

Howard, Jane K., and Jeffrey S. Flier. 2006. "Attenuation of Leptin and Insulin Signaling by SOCS Proteins." *Trends in Endocrinology & Metabolism* 17 (9): 365–71. https://doi.org/10.1016/j.tem.2006.09.007.

Howell, Kristy R., and Theresa L. Powell. 2017. "Effects of Maternal Obesity on Placental Function and Fetal Development." *Reproduction* 153 (3): R97–108. https://doi.org/10.1530/REP-16-0495.

Hribal, Marta, Teresa Fiorentino, and Giorgio Sesti. 2014. "Role of C Reactive Protein (CRP) in Leptin Resistance." *Current Pharmaceutical Design* 20 (4): 609–15. https://doi.org/10.2174/13816128113199990016.

Jiang, Mengqi, Jianyi He, Yingxu Sun, Xin Dong, Jiayu Yao, Hailun Gu, and Li Liu. 2021. "Leptin Induced TLR4 Expression via the JAK2-STAT3 Pathway in Obesity-Related Osteoarthritis." Edited by Kai Wang. *Oxidative Medicine and Cellular Longevity* 2021 (August): 1–16. https://doi.org/10.1155/2021/7385160.

Kamareddine, Layla, Crystal M. Ghantous, Soumaya Allouch, Sarah A. Al-Ashmar, Gulsen Anlar, Surya Kannan, Laiche Djouhri, Hesham M. Korashy, Abdelali Agouni, and Asad Zeidan. 2021. "Between Inflammation and Autophagy: The Role of Leptin-Adiponectin Axis in Cardiac Remodeling." *Journal of Inflammation Research* Volume 14 (October): 5349–65. https://doi.org/10.2147/JIR.S322231.

Kiernan, Kaitlin, and Nancie J. MacIver. 2021. "The Role of the Adipokine Leptin in Immune Cell Function in Health and Disease." *Frontiers in Immunology* 11 (January). https://doi.org/10.3389/fimmu.2020.622468.

Kim, Min-Hyun, and Hyeyoung Kim. 2021. "Role of Leptin in the Digestive System." *Frontiers in Pharmacology* 12 (April). https://doi.org/10.3389/fphar.2021.660040.

Korczynska, Justyna, Aleksandra Czumaj, Michal Chmielewski, Julian Swierczynski, and Tomasz Sledzinski. 2021. "The Causes and Potential Injurious Effects of Elevated Serum Leptin Levels in Chronic Kidney Disease Patients." *International Journal of Molecular Sciences* 22 (9): 4685. https://doi.org/10.3390/ijms22094685.

Landry, David A., François Sormany, Josée Haché, Pauline Roumaud, and Luc J. Martin. 2017. "Steroidogenic Genes Expressions Are Repressed by High Levels of Leptin and the JAK/STAT Signaling Pathway in MA-10 Leydig Cells." *Molecular and Cellular Biochemistry* 433 (1–2): 79–95. https://doi.org/10.1007/s11010-017-3017-x.

Lin, Tsung-Chieh, and Michael Hsiao. 2021. "Leptin and Cancer: Updated Functional Roles in Carcinogenesis, Therapeutic Niches, and Developments." *International Journal of Molecular Sciences* 22 (6): 2870. https://doi.org/10.3390/ijms22062870.

Luque, Raul M., Zhi H. Huang, Bhumik Shah, Theodore Mazzone, and Rhonda D. Kineman. 2007. "Effects of Leptin Replacement on Hypothalamic-Pituitary Growth Hormone Axis Function and Circulating Ghrelin Levels in Ob/Ob Mice." *American Journal of Physiology-Endocrinology and Metabolism* 292 (3): E891–99. https://doi.org/10.1152/ajpendo.00258.2006.

Madeddu, Clelia, Elisabetta Sanna, Giulia Gramignano, Luciana Tanca, Maria Cristina Cherchi, Brunella Mola, Marco Petrillo, and Antonio Macciò. 2022. "Correlation of Leptin, Proinflammatory Cytokines and Oxidative Stress with Tumor Size and Disease Stage of Endometrioid (Type I) Endometrial Cancer and Review of the Underlying Mechanisms." *Cancers* 14 (2): 268. https://doi.org/10.3390/cancers14020268.

Martínez-Sánchez, Noelia. 2020. "There and Back Again: Leptin Actions in White Adipose Tissue." *International Journal of Molecular Sciences* 21 (17): 6039. https://doi.org/10.3390/ijms21176039.

Martínez-Uña, Maite, Yaiza López-Mancheño, Carlos Diéguez, Manuel A. Fernández-Rojo, and Marta G. Novelle. 2020. "Unraveling the Role of Leptin in Liver Function and Its Relationship with Liver Diseases." *International Journal of Molecular Sciences* 21 (24): 9368. https://doi.org/10.3390/ijms21249368.

Maurya, Radheshyam, Parna Bhattacharya, Ranadhir Dey, and Hira L Nakhasi. 2018. "Leptin Functions in Infectious Diseases." *Frontiers in Immunology* 9 (November): 2741. https://doi.org/10.3389/fimmu.2018.02741.

Maymó, Julieta L., Antonio Pérez Pérez, José L. Dueñas, Juan Carlos Calvo, Víctor Sánchez-Margalet, and Cecilia L Varone. 2010. "Regulation of Placental Leptin Expression by Cyclic Adenosine 5′-Monophosphate Involves Cross Talk between Protein Kinase A and Mitogen-Activated Protein Kinase Signaling Pathways." *Endocrinology* 151 (8): 3738–51. https://doi.org/10.1210/en.2010-0064.

Maymó, Julieta Lorena, Antonio Pérez Pérez, Bernardo Maskin, José Luis Dueñas, Juan Carlos Calvo, Víctor Sánchez Margalet, and Cecilia Laura Varone. 2012. "The Alternative Epac/CAMP Pathway and the MAPK Pathway Mediate HCG Induction of Leptin in Placental Cells." Edited by Tamas Zakar. *PLoS ONE* 7 (10): e46216. https://doi.org/10.1371/journal.pone.0046216.

Mendoza-Herrera, Kenny, Andrea A. Florio, Maggie Moore, Abrania Marrero, Martha Tamez, Shilpa N. Bhupathiraju, and Josiemer Mattei. 2021. "The Leptin System and Diet: A Mini Review of the Current Evidence." *Frontiers in Endocrinology* 12 (November). https://doi.org/10.3389/fendo.2021.749050.

Milling, Simon. 2019. "Adipokines and the Control of Mast Cell Functions: From Obesity to Inflammation?" *Immunology* 158 (1): 1–2. https://doi.org/10.1111/imm.13104.

Mullen, McKay, and Ruben Gonzalez-Perez. 2016. "Leptin-Induced JAK/STAT Signaling and Cancer Growth." *Vaccines* 4 (3): 26. https://doi.org/10.3390/vaccines4030026.

Mullur, Rashmi, Yan-Yun Liu, and Gregory A. Brent. 2014. "Thyroid Hormone Regulation of Metabolism." *Physiological Reviews* 94 (2): 355–82. https://doi.org/10.1152/physrev.00030.2013.

Naylor, Caitlin, and William A. Petri. 2016. "Leptin Regulation of Immune Responses." *Trends in Molecular Medicine* 22 (2): 88–98. https://doi.org/10.1016/j.molmed.2015.12.001.

Neelamekam, Sasi, Milawaty Nurjono, and Jimmy Lee. 2014. "Regulation of Interleukin-6 and Leptin in Schizophrenia Patients: A Preliminary Analysis." *Clinical Psychopharmacology and Neuroscience* 12 (3): 209–14. https://doi.org/10.9758/cpn.2014.12.3.209.

Nillni, Eduardo A. 2010. "Regulation of the Hypothalamic Thyrotropin Releasing Hormone (TRH) Neuron by Neuronal and Peripheral Inputs." *Frontiers in Neuroendocrinology* 31 (2): 134–56. https://doi.org/10.1016/j.yfrne.2010.01.001.

Park, Hyeong-Kyu, and Rexford S. Ahima. 2015. "Physiology of Leptin: Energy Homeostasis, Neuroendocrine Function and Metabolism." *Metabolism* 64 (1): 24–34. https://doi.org/10.1016/j.metabol.2014.08.004.

Patraca, Iván, Nohora Martínez, Oriol Busquets, Aleix Martí, Ignacio Pedrós, Carlos Beas-Zarate, Miguel Marin, Ettcheto, M., Sureda, F., Auladell, C., Camins, A., & Folch, J. 2017. "Anti-Inflammatory Role of Leptin in Glial Cells through P38 MAPK Pathway Inhibition." *Pharmacological Reports* 69 (3): 409–18. https://doi.org/10.1016/j.pharep.2016.12.005.

Pérez-Pérez, Antonio, Flora Sánchez-Jiménez, Teresa Vilariño-García, and Víctor Sánchez-Margalet. 2020. "Role of Leptin in Inflammation and Vice Versa." *International Journal of Molecular Sciences* 21 (16): 5887. https://doi.org/10.3390/ijms21165887.

Pertiwi, Kartika R., Onno J. de Boer, Claire Mackaaij, Dara R. Pabittei, Robbert J. de Winter, Xiaofei Li, and Allard C. van der Wal. 2019. "Extracellular Traps Derived from Macrophages, Mast Cells, Eosinophils and Neutrophils Are Generated in a Time-Dependent Manner during Atherothrombosis." *The Journal of Pathology* 247 (4): 505–12. https://doi.org/10.1002/path.5212.

Piessevaux, Julie, Delphine Lavens, Tony Montoye, Joris Wauman, Dominiek Catteeuw, Joël Vandekerckhove, Denise Belsham, Frank Peelman, and Jan Tavernier. 2006.

"Functional Cross-Modulation between SOCS Proteins Can Stimulate Cytokine Signaling." *Journal of Biological Chemistry* 281 (44): 32953–66. https://doi.org/10.1074/jbc.M600776200.

Procaccini, Claudio, Emilio Jirillo, and Giuseppe Matarese. 2012. "Leptin as an Immunomodulator." *Molecular Aspects of Medicine* 33 (1): 35–45. https://doi.org/10.1016/j.mam.2011.10.012.

Rehman, Kanwal, Muhammad Sajid Hamid Akash, and Zunaira Alina. 2018. "Leptin: A New Therapeutic Target for Treatment of Diabetes Mellitus." *Journal of Cellular Biochemistry* 119 (7): 5016–27. https://doi.org/10.1002/jcb.26580.

Rosa, Salvatore De, Plinio Cirillo, Mario Pacileo, Vito Di Palma, Antonella Paglia, and Massimo Chiariello. 2009. "Leptin Stimulated C-Reactive Protein Production by Human Coronary Artery Endothelial Cells." *Journal of Vascular Research* 46 (6): 609–17. https://doi.org/10.1159/000226229.

Safai, Narges, Stefanie Eising, David Michael Hougaard, Henrik Bindesbøl Mortensen, Kristin Skogstrand, Flemming Pociot, Jesper Johannesen, and Jannet Svensson. 2015. "Levels of Adiponectin and Leptin at Onset of Type 1 Diabetes Have Changed over Time in Children and Adolescents." *Acta Diabetologica* 52 (1): 167–74. https://doi.org/10.1007/s00592-014-0630-y.

Salazar, Juan, Mervin Chávez-Castillo, Joselyn Rojas, Angel Ortega, Manuel Nava, José Pérez, Milagros Rojas, D'Marco, L., & Bermudez, V. 2020. "Is 'Leptin Resistance' Another Key Resistance to Manage Type 2 Diabetes?" *Current Diabetes Reviews* 16 (7): 733–49. https://doi.org/10.2174/1573399816666191230111838.

Saleri, Roberta, Andrea Giustina, Carlo Tamanini, Domenico Valle, Anna Burattin, William B. Wehrenberg, and Mario Baratta. 2004. "Leptin Stimulates Growth Hormone Secretion via a Direct Pituitary Effect Combined with a Decreased Somatostatin Tone in a Median Eminence-Pituitary Perifusion Study." *Neuroendocrinology* 79 (4): 221–28. https://doi.org/10.1159/000078103.

Scabia, Gaia, Ilaria Barone, Marco Mainardi, Giovanni Ceccarini, Manuela Scali, Emma Buzzigoli, Alessia Dattilo, Vitti, P., Gastaldelli, A., Santini, F., Pizzorusso, T., Maffei, L., & Maffei, M. 2018. "The Antidepressant Fluoxetine Acts on Energy Balance and Leptin Sensitivity via BDNF." *Scientific Reports* 8 (1): 1781. https://doi.org/10.1038/s41598-018-19886-x.

Shapses, Sue A., L. Claudia Pop, and Yang Wang. 2017. "Obesity Is a Concern for Bone Health with Aging." *Nutrition Research* 39 (March): 1–13. https://doi.org/10.1016/j.nutres.2016.12.010.

Singh, Prachi, Michal Hoffmann, Robert Wolk, Abu S. M. Shamsuzzaman, and Virend K. Somers. 2007. "Leptin Induces C-Reactive Protein Expression in Vascular Endothelial Cells." *Arteriosclerosis, Thrombosis, and Vascular Biology* 27 (9). https://doi.org/10.1161/ATVBAHA.107.148353.

Souza-Almeida, Glaucia, Lohanna Palhinha, Sally Liechocki, Jéssica Aparecida da Silva Pereira, Patrícia Alves Reis, Paula Ribeiro Braga Dib, Eugenio D. Hottz, Gameiro, J., Vallochi, A. L., De Almeida, C. J., Castro-Faria-Neto, H., Bozza, P. T., & Maya-Monteiro, C. M. 2021. "Peripheral Leptin Signaling Persists in Innate Immune Cells during Diet-Induced Obesity." *Journal of Leukocyte Biology* 109 (6): 1131–38. https://doi.org/10.1002/JLB.3AB0820-092RR.

Sutton, Amy K., Martin G. Myers, and David P. Olson. 2016. "The Role of PVH Circuits in Leptin Action and Energy Balance." *Annual Review of Physiology* 78 (1): 207–21. https://doi.org/10.1146/annurev-physiol-021115-105347.

Tanida, Mamoru, Naoki Yamamoto, Donald A. Morgan, Yasutaka Kurata, Toshishige Shibamoto, and Kamal Rahmouni. 2015. "Leptin Receptor Signaling in the Hypothalamus Regulates Hepatic Autonomic Nerve Activity via Phosphatidylinositol 3-Kinase and AMP-Activated Protein Kinase." *The Journal of Neuroscience* 35 (2): 474–84. https://doi.org/10.1523/JNEUROSCI.1828-14.2015.

Tazawa, Ryo, Kentaro Uchida, Hisako Fujimaki, Masayuki Miyagi, Gen Inoue, Hiroyuki Sekiguchi, Kosuke Murata, Ken Takata, Ayumu Kawakubo, and Masashi Takaso. 2019. "Elevated Leptin Levels Induce Inflammation through IL-6 in Skeletal Muscle of Aged Female Rats." *BMC Musculoskeletal Disorders* 20 (1): 1–7. https://doi.org/10.1186/S12891-019-2581-5/FIGURES/4.

Thiagarajan, Praveena S., Qiao Zheng, Manvir Bhagrath, Erin E. Mulkearns-Hubert, Martin G. Myers, Justin D. Lathia, and Ofer Reizes. 2017. "STAT3 Activation by Leptin Receptor Is Essential for TNBC Stem Cell Maintenance." *Endocrine-Related Cancer* 24 (8): 415–26. https://doi.org/10.1530/ERC-16-0349.

Torchen, Laura, Beth Hakamy, Margaret Sullivan, Erica E Marsh, and Lisa M Neff. 2022. "RF24 | PSUN127 Congenital Leptin Deficiency: Metabolic, Reproductive, and Psychological Impacts of Therapy." *Journal of the Endocrine Society* 6 (Supplement_1): A34–35. https://doi.org/10.1210/jendso/bvac150.072.

Torpy, D., S. Bornstein, and G. Chrousos. 1998. "Leptin and Interleukin-6 in Sepsis." *Hormone and Metabolic Research* 30 (12): 726–29. https://doi.org/10.1055/s-2007-978967.

Tsuchiya, Haruka, and Keishi Fujio. 2022. "Emerging Role of Leptin in Joint Inflammation and Destruction." *Immunological Medicine* 45 (1): 27–34. https://doi.org/10.1080/25785826.2021.1948689.

Uchiyama, Takashi, Hirokazu Takahashi, Michiko Sugiyama, Eiji Sakai, Hiroki Endo, Kunihiro Hosono, Kyoko Yoneda, Inamori, M., Nagashima, Y., Inayama, Y., Wada, K., & Nakajima, A. 2011. "Leptin Receptor Is Involved in STAT3 Activation in Human Colorectal Adenoma." *Cancer Science* 102 (2): 367–72. https://doi.org/10.1111/j.1349-7006.2010.01803.x.

Upadhyay, Jagriti, Olivia M. Farr, and Christos S. Mantzoros. 2015. "The Role of Leptin in Regulating Bone Metabolism." *Metabolism* 64 (1): 105–13. https://doi.org/10.1016/J.METABOL.2014.10.021.

Viikari, Liisa A., Risto K. Huupponen, Jorma S. A. Viikari, Jukka Marniemi, Carita Eklund, Mikko Hurme, Terho Lehtimäki, Mika Kivimäki, and Olli T. Raitakari. 2007. "Relationship between Leptin and C-Reactive Protein in Young Finnish Adults." *The Journal of Clinical Endocrinology & Metabolism* 92 (12): 4753–58. https://doi.org/10.1210/jc.2007-0103.

Wauters, M., RV Considine, and LF Van Gaal. 2000. "Human Leptin: From an Adipocyte Hormone to an Endocrine Mediator." *European Journal of Endocrinology* 143 (3): 293–311. https://doi.org/10.1530/eje.0.1430293.

Yang, Wei-Hung, Shan-Chi Liu, Chun-Hao Tsai, Yi-Chin Fong, Shoou-Jyi Wang, Yung-Sen Chang, and Chih-Hsin Tang. 2013. "Leptin Induces IL-6 Expression through

OBRl Receptor Signaling Pathway in Human Synovial Fibroblasts." Edited by Victor Sanchez-Margalet. *PLoS ONE* 8 (9): e75551. https://doi.org/10.1371/journal.pone.0075551.

Yi, Xuejie, Haining Gao, Dequan Chen, Donghui Tang, Wanting Huang, Tao Li, Tie Ma, and Bo Chang. 2017. "Effects of Obesity and Exercise on Testicular Leptin Signal Transduction and Testosterone Biosynthesis in Male Mice." *American Journal of Physiology-Regulatory, Integrative and Comparative Physiology* 312 (4): R501–10. https://doi.org/10.1152/ajpregu.00405.2016.

Yupanqui-Lozno, Hernan, Raul A. Bastarrachea, Maria E. Yupanqui-Velazco, Monica Alvarez-Jaramillo, Esteban Medina-Méndez, Aida P. Giraldo-Peña, Alexandra Arias-Serrano, Torres-Forero, C., Garcia-Ordoñez, A. M., Mastronardi, C. A., Restrepo, C. M., Rodriguez-Ayala, E., Nava-Gonzalez, E. J., Arcos-Burgos, M., Kent, J. W., Cole, S. A., Licinio, J., & Celis-Regalado, L. G. 2019. "Congenital Leptin Deficiency and Leptin Gene Missense Mutation Found in Two Colombian Sisters with Severe Obesity." *Genes* 10 (5): 342. https://doi.org/10.3390/genes10050342.

Zarrati, Mitra, Nahid Aboutaleb, Elhameh Cheshmazar, Raheleh Shokouhi Shoormasti, Elham Razmpoosh, and Farinaz Nasirinezhad. 2019. "The Association of Obesity and Serum Leptin Levels with Complete Blood Count and Some Serum Biochemical Parameters in Iranian Overweight and Obese Individuals." *Medical Journal of the Islamic Republic of Iran* 33 (1): 72. https://doi.org/10.34171/mjiri.33.72.

Zhang, Faming, Yanyun Chen, Mark Heiman, and Richard DiMarchi. 2005. "Leptin: Structure, Function and Biology." In *Vitamins and Hormones*, 71:345–72. Academic Press. https://doi.org/10.1016/S0083-6729(05)71012-8.

Zhang, Yiying, and Streamson Chua. 2017. "Leptin Function and Regulation." In *Comprehensive Physiology*, 8:351–69. Wiley. https://doi.org/10.1002/cphy.c160041.

Zimmerman, Arthur D., and Ruth B. S. Harris. 2015. "*In Vivo* and *in Vitro* Evidence That Chronic Activation of the Hexosamine Biosynthetic Pathway Interferes with Leptin-Dependent STAT3 Phosphorylation." *American Journal of Physiology-Regulatory, Integrative and Comparative Physiology* 308 (6): R543–55. https://doi.org/10.1152/ajpregu.00347.2014.

Chapter 3

The Effects of Leptin on the Cardiovascular System

Ümit Kılıç[1], PhD
Hayriye Soytürk[2,*], PhD
Eylem Suveren[3], PhD
and Ayşcgül Yıldız[4], PhD

[1]Duzce University Vocational School of Health Services, Duzce, Turkey
[2]Bolu Abant Izzet Baysal University, Institute of Graduate Studies Interdisciplinary Neuroscience, Bolu, Turkey
[3]Bolu Abant Izzet Baysal University, Faculty of Health Sciences, Department of Nursing, Bolu, Turkey
[4]Bolu Abant Izzet Baysal University, Medical School, Department of Physiology Bolu, Turkey

Abstract

Leptin hormone is an adipokine released from adipose tissue that has recently gained interest due to its impact on the cardiovascular system as well as many other systemic effects. The obesity (ob) gene regulates leptin hormone release, which plays a role in body fat regulation. Obesity, which is defined by a rise in blood leptin levels, is a key risk factor for cardiovascular disease. Because of the increased activity of the sympathetic nervous system and the accompanying renin-angiotensin system, obesity produces a rise in extracellular fluid volume. The increase in sympathetic activity caused by hyperleptinemia is one of the reasons for obesity-related hypertension. One of the reasons for

---

* Corresponding Author's Email: hayriyesoyturk1@gmail.com.

In: Leptin and its Role in Health and Disease
Editor: Stephen E. Bradley
ISBN: 979-8-89113-274-0
© 2024 Nova Science Publishers, Inc.

cardiovascular diseases in obesity is the interplay of angiotensin II, insulin, endothelin-A, and hyperleptinemia. Acute cardiovascular events, restenosis following coronary angioplasty, and cerebral palsy have all been linked to high leptin levels. In leptin-deficient mice, arterial thrombosis was shown to be minimal. As a result, inhibiting leptin activation could be a future therapy method for hyperleptinemic obese people to reduce the course of atherosclerosis.

This book chapter will discuss the consequences of hyperleptinemia caused by high leptin serum levels and leptin receptor resistance in obesity on renal, cardiac, vascular, and sympathetic nervous system function, as well as their relationship to cardiovascular disease.

Keywords: leptin, hypertension, cardiovascular diseases, obesity, sympathetic nervous system

Introduction

Obesity-related comorbidities such as type 2 diabetes mellitus, dyslipidemia, fatty liver disease, hypertension, heart disease, and some types of cancer kill around 3.4 million people each year, according to World Health Organization data. (World Health Organization; (2019)

Obesity is a chronic metabolic disorder. Obesity-related hypertension, atherosclerosis, cardiac hypertrophy, diabetes, and dyslipidemia all increase the risk of developing cardiovascular and metabolic disorders (Despres JP 2006; Van Gaal, Mertens, and De Block 2006).

The relationships between obesity and cardiovascular disease, however, are not entirely understood. Leptin has been proven in numerous studies to have direct effects on the cardiovascular system. Adipocytes, as well as the heart, vascular smooth muscle, placenta, and digestive epithelium, produce leptin. As a result, leptin is assumed to play an essential role in the relationship between obesity and cardiovascular disease.

Understanding how leptin affects the cardiovascular system will provide insight into the cardiovascular consequences of obesity. This article highlights the current understanding of the association between leptin and cardiovascular disease.

The Structure of Leptin and the Mechanism of Leptin Signaling

Leptin is a peptide hormone that white adipose tissue produces. The leptin (LEP or OB) gene is located on chromosome 7q31.3.4.(Gong et al. 1996) The mature protein has 146 amino acids and is created by protein synthesis for mRNA (Wasim et al. 2016). Leptin is a 16-kDa hormone produced by the OB gene that is essential for regulating energy homeostasis. Obesity results from a lack of leptin, which causes increased appetite and decreased energy expenditure. Obesity in children, on the other hand, has rarely been documented as a result of leptin insufficiency. Most overweight people have much higher serum leptin levels than their normal-weight counterparts (Wallace et al. 2001).

In obese people and animal models, high circulating leptin levels have been linked to total body fat mass. This is believed to be due to leptin resistance. Leptin resembles proinflammatory cytokines prevalent in the body, such as interleukin 6 and granulocyte colony-stimulating factor, in structure (Peelman et al. 2014). The concentration of leptin in the blood is related to the quantity of adipose tissue. Leptin exerts its action on the cell surface by attaching to leptin receptors (LR). Neuronal, hepatic, pancreatic, cardiac, and perivascular intestinal tissues contain leptin receptors (Dornbush S 2023).

According to current knowledge, the Janus-activated kinase/signal transducers and activators of transcription (Jak/STAT), mitogen-activated protein kinases (MAPK), and phosphatidylinositol 3-kinase (PI-3K) signaling pathways primarily modify the leptin signaling route.

Leptin and Its Receptors and Molecular Mechanisms of Leptin

Adipocytes are the cells that create leptin. It is released at a faster rate in the early morning and late evening. Although leptin release occurs independently of mRNA regulation (Sinha et al. 1996), greater leptin mRNA transcription is essential to maintain steady rates of leptin secretion and prevent leptin vesicle depletion. Leptin circulates in the serum in both free and bound forms once it is secreted (Ye et al. 2010). These receptors are the hypothalamus, pancreas, ovary, testis, uterus, kidney, heart, lung, liver, adrenal gland, hematopoietic stem cells, and skeletal muscles have all been discovered to contain it. LEPRa,

LEPRb, LEPRc, LEPRd, LEPRe, and LEPRf are the six isoforms of leptin receptors (Ahima and Osei 2004).

LR is a cytokine receptor that belongs to the glycoprotein 130 family and has six isoforms. Isoform-b is the most well-studied of these isoforms. The receptor subtype that predominantly facilitates the activation of essential second messenger pathways and proper leptin function is the long form (Allison and Myers 2014). The JAK-STAT signaling route is the primary LR signaling pathway. Leptin binds to LR, causing it to dimerize.

The JAK2 tyrosine kinase is activated as a result of this dimerization, and it phosphorylates three tyrosine residues that serve as docking sites for the SHP2, STAT5, and STAT3 proteins. SHP's role is to participate in the ERK signal. Stat5's function has yet to be discovered. Stat 3 is a transcription factor that is responsible for modulating leptin's principal activities (Dornbush S 2023).

Leptin Secretion Regulation

Leptin's primary site of action is the brain, particularly the brain stem and hypothalamus. The solitary system and the ventral tegmental region are the primary sites of action in the brainstem. The major areas of action of leptin in the hypothalamus include the lateral hypothalamic area and the ventromedial, dorsomedial, ventral premammillary, and arcuate (ARC) nuclei (Amjad et al. 2019; Farr, Olivia M, Gavirieli 2017). The most well-known of them is leptin's effect on the ARC nucleus. The ARC core is crucial in regulating appetite and energy homeostasis. It consists of orexigenic agouti-associated protein/neuropeptide Y (AgRP/NPY) neurons and anorexigenic proopiomelanocortin (POMC) neurons. Leptin suppresses hunger by activating POMC-containing neurons and inhibiting AgRP/NPY-containing neurons in the ARC nucleus (Dornbush S 2023).

As the size of adipose tissue reduces, so does the amount of leptin generated and crossing the blood-brain barrier. The CNS stops the decline in leptin as a signal of a lack of energy, triggering a cascade of responses to assist the body in coping with the stress of hunger. To compensate for a lack of energy, the CNS not only increases hunger but also promotes energy-saving autonomic strategies such as lowered neuroendocrine and sympathetic nervous system tone, thyroid and reproductive hormone levels, energy expenditure, and development. A drop in serum leptin is a hunger signal to the CNS. As the intake of food rises and the amount of adipose tissue increases, leptin synthesis and release into the bloodstream rise as well. Increased leptin inhibits appetite, resulting in lower food intake and higher energy expenditure to balance the available energy surplus (Dornbush S 2023).

A fully functional leptin system is present in all areas of the heart, including leptin production and the fully functional long form of its receptor (Purdham et al. 2004). As a result, leptin signaling is critical for maintaining proper cardiac function. There is a beneficial inverse connection between carotid wall thickness and measures of circulating leptin in healthy young men, suggesting leptin's vascular protective effect (Ahiante et al. 2019).

Human Leptin Studies

Although rare, congenital leptin insufficiency in humans may reveal crucial information regarding the role of leptin. Genetic mutations in both the leptin gene and the leptin receptor gene have been found, and both genetic variants induce similar phenotypes in terms of immune response. Mutations in the leptin or leptin receptor gene cause early-onset severe obesity, hyperphagia, hypogonadism, and metabolic problems (Nunziata et al. 2019). Furthermore, these patients get recurring infections, and those with leptin insufficiency are in danger of dying from intracellular infections (Ozata, Ozdemir, and Licinio 1999). Leptin replacement therapy has been found to boost CD4 T cell counts in humans and reverse abnormalities in CD4 T cell proliferation and cytokine production (Sadaf Farooqi et al. 2002). These findings demonstrate the significance of leptin's inappropriate immune function and infection prevention. Fasting lowers leptin levels and results in lower blood lymphocyte numbers, which is consistent with this (Chan et al. 2006).

While the pathophysiology of obesity is multifaceted, elevated leptin signaling may produce excessive inflammation and a cytokine storm (Kiernan and MacIver 2021).

Leptin and Cardiovascular Disease Animal Models

Animal models have aided in the understanding of leptin signaling in the heart(Boudina and Abel 2007), and both ob/ob and db/db mice exhibit age-related hypertrophy, primarily impacting left ventricular (LV) mass and AG wall thickness (Barouch et al. 2003; Yue et al. 2007).

Under physiological settings, the heart uses both glucose and free fatty acids as energy sources. In rodent models lacking leptin or LR, cardiac performance is impaired, vesicular fatty acid uptake is increased, and glucose uptake is decreased, and this is associated with altered myocardial substrate uptake and metabolic inelasticity due to carbohydrate oxidation and fatty acid oxidation.

Because glucose is a more efficient energy substrate for cardiomyocytes than free fatty acids, switching from glucose metabolism to free fatty acid oxidation results in systemic metabolic disorders characterized by increased myocardial oxygen consumption (MVO2) and decreased cardiac efficiency (ratio of cardiac work to energy input) (Golfman et al. 2005; Buchanan et al. 2005). Animals lacking leptin or LR have higher triglyceride levels and accumulation of lipids in the heart, which may induce lipotoxicity and decrease cardiac contractility (Sharma et al. 2004).

This shows that Leptin may operate as an anti-lipotoxic adipokine, protecting the heart from damaging lipid accumulation and the advancement of cardiac steatosis, especially under cardiac stress. Using leptin- or LR-deficient mouse models, researchers discovered that leptin works as a metabolic, cardioprotective adipokine, especially under ischemic conditions (Poetsch, Strano, and Guan 2020).

Pathophysiology

Leptin deficiency or resistance is associated with dysregulation of cytokine production, increased susceptibility to infections, autoimmune disorders, malnutrition, and inflammatory responses.

Hypoleptinemia

Leptin deficiency results in clinical phenotypes of severe obesity, impaired satiety, intense hyperphagia, persistent foraging behavior, recurrent bacterial infections, hyperinsulinemia, fatty liver, dyslipidemia, and hypogonadotropic hypogonadism (Funcke et al. 2014; Sadaf Farooqi and O'Rahilly 2014).

These phenotypes demonstrate the various roles leptin plays in the body, many of which are still being studied but are not fully understood. Congenital hypoleptinemia is caused by LEP or LR gene abnormalities and is referred to as congenital leptin deficiency (CLD). Appropriate leptin signaling is required for good cardiac performance. Leptin deficiency has been linked to cardiovascular problems in rat models of lipodystrophy and leptin deficiency (Dong et al. 2006; Mazumder et al. 2004; Zhao, Kusminski, and Scherer 2021). Hyperleptinemia, on the other hand, which is common in diet-induced obesity, causes cardiovascular problems and increases death rates. To target a leptin-based therapy for cardiovascular illnesses, one should concentrate on circulating leptin levels. In the case of total leptin deficit, leptin treatment (raising leptin levels to physiological levels) is adequate to prevent or reverse cardiovascular disease.

The use of meter leptin (a recombinant version of leptin) to treat lipodystrophy patients is well established. More particular, leptin treatment significantly normalizes glucose tolerance and insulin sensitivity in these lipodystrophic people, improving liver and cardiac function (Arioglu et al. 2002).

However, leptin treatment is typically unsuccessful in the context of hyperleptinemia. Instead, reducing circulating leptin levels to attain a normal systemic range has significant promise in the treatment of obesity and its accompanying cardiovascular diseases. It should be highlighted in this regard that this strategy does not necessitate sophisticated titration to normalize leptin levels. Metabolic researchers have identified a broad therapeutic range for leptin neutralization therapy. Any considerable reduction in leptin levels results in favorable effects, i.e., leptin levels can be drastically reduced while still reaping the benefits (Zhao, Kusminski, and Scherer 2021).

Hyperleptinemia

Leptin resistance is linked to hyperleptinemia. Obesity is characterized by hyperleptinemia and leptin resistance. This relationship is explained by a direct link between blood leptin concentrations and body fat percentage, with obese people having higher leptin serum levels and adipocyte LEP mRNA content than average-weight people. Furthermore, as weight is lost, leptin blood levels and adipocyte LEP mRNA content decline. Resistance appears to be caused by impairments in leptin trafficking across the blood-brain barrier or intracellular signaling systems downstream of the LR. Nonalcoholic fatty liver disease, Rabson-Mendenhall syndrome, neurodegenerative illnesses, depression, and food addiction are among the diseases associated with hyperleptinemia (Peters et al. 2018).

Researchers have discovered that hyperleptinemia alone is sufficient to increase leptin resistance. Obesity and its related metabolic problems are exacerbated by high leptin levels. This raised the prospect of reducing circulating leptin levels as an effective treatment for obesity and its metabolic implications (Zhao, Kusminski, et al. 2020). This has been established in investigations using leptin-neutralizing antibodies as well as genetic mouse models. Partially decreasing leptin restores leptin's physiological role in reducing food intake and raising energy expenditure, leading to significant weight loss and anti-diabetic effects. Based on these data, we hypothesize that partial leptin suppression will also ameliorate the etiology of cardiovascular dysfunction, hence improving the outcome of a cardiovascular event (Zhao, Kusminski, and Scherer 2021).

Obesity-related CVD is associated with increased leptin levels, according to observational evidence (Abe et al. 2007). Several large population-based studies have demonstrated strong positive relationships between high leptin levels and cardiovascular problems such as hypertension, diabetes, coronary heart disease, and stroke in various populations. Suggested (Welsh et al. 2009; Liu et al. 2010).

Many observations have indirectly indicated the effectiveness of partial leptin decrease in the context of hyperleptinemia. Lifestyle adjustments and pharmacological therapies that promote cardiovascular health are linked to a decrease in circulating leptin levels. Long-term calorie restriction, for example, protects heart contractile activity, which improves cardiomyocyte function and reduces cardiac remodeling (Shinmura et al. 2011; Han et al. 2012).

Calorie restriction also successfully lowers leptin levels in the blood (Robertson et al. 2015; Rogozina OP, Bonorden MJ, Seppanen CN 2011). High-intensity physical activity has also been demonstrated to reduce leptin levels while improving cardiovascular function (Racil et al. 2016). Lowering circulating leptin levels in the context of hyperleptinemia may thus directly contribute to cardiovascular improvements (Zhao, Kusminski, and Scherer 2021).

Cardiovascular Diseases and Leptin

The role of leptin in the cardiovascular system remains debatable. According to numerous studies, leptin has a function in the etiology of chronic inflammation. In this context, it is thought that increased leptin levels in obese patients contribute to low-grade systemic inflammation, making obese people more vulnerable to cardiovascular disease. Furthermore, higher leptin levels in patients with dilated cardiomyopathy have been documented, and this has been employed as a biomarker for the progression of heart failure independent of immunological responses (Bobbert et al. 2012).

There is currently no valid model to explain the seemingly contradictory effects of leptin on cardiovascular function. Recent findings on the impact of leptin on body weight regulation provide a novel way to explain these paradoxical effects on the cardiovascular system. Lowering circulating leptin levels results in a large increase in food intake and body weight gain in the setting of leptin sensitivity, which is most noticeable in young and thin mice. This is consistent with previous models that describe the response to reduced leptin levels. In cases of leptin resistance, however, a distinct reaction is observed. A partial leptin reduction causes increased leptin sensitivity, enhanced insulin sensitivity, and a drop in body weight (Zhao, Kusminski, et al. 2020; Zhao, Li, et al. 2020). This seemingly contradictory reaction to leptin reduction in the overall domain of weight maintenance and energy expenditure may also be essential to a better understanding of leptin's contradictory effects on cardiovascular function. Furthermore, hyperleptinemia is sufficient in obesogenic settings to promote spontaneous leptin resistance, resulting in all other metabolic diseases commonly associated with weight gain.

Thus, in the first approach, circulating leptin levels represent the status of an individual's leptin sensitivity: more circulating leptin translates to lower leptin sensitivity. Based on these findings, the researchers suggest a new paradigm in which properly sustained leptin signaling over a narrow range is required for good cardiac function.

These findings highlight the paradoxical repercussions of leptin-related actions on the cardiovascular system; that is, both excess exogenous leptin and leptin shortage frequently result in cardiovascular dysfunction. More research is needed to determine whether these effects are caused by wholly different processes or are mediated by various Ob-R isoform rearrangements. These distinctions can be reconciled in particular if we consider both leptin shortage and leptin resistance to be states of downstream signaling failure (Hou and Luo 2011).

Obesity-related chronic hyperleptinemia/selective leptin central resistance contributes to the development of cardiovascular illnesses such as hypertension, cardiac hypertrophy and remodeling, atherosclerosis, and heart failure (Hou and Luo 2011).

Dysfunction of the Endothelium

Hypertension, atherosclerosis, and coronary artery disease are all caused by endothelial dysfunction. Endothelial dysfunction is frequently regarded as a risk factor for atherosclerosis disease. Although there is evidence that leptin mediates this process, it is important to note that endothelial dysfunction is often detected at supraphysiological doses (Korda et al. 2008).

Endothelial dysfunction caused by leptin is related to increased oxidative stress and decreased NO bioavailability. Several studies have found that mice treated with leptin have higher levels of oxidative stress indicators as well as lower levels of antioxidant molecules (Bełtowski, Wójcicka, and Jamroz 2003). Although leptin has a direct vasodilatory impact by promoting NO generation, the acute effects of leptin may differ significantly from the long-term increase. Korda et al. discovered that prolonged (12-hour) leptin treatment lowers bioavailable NO despite a two-fold increase in endothelial NO synthase (eNOS) expression. This causes a NO/ONOO imbalance, which impairs endothelial function (Korda et al. 2008).

Leptin, Cardiac Fibrosis and Vascular Dysfunction

Leptin-mediated production of aldosterone is considered a novel mechanism of obesity-associated endothelial dysfunction and cardiac fibrosis, impairing myocardial relaxation and thus contributing to cardiovascular disease (Huby et al. 2015). Correlation between leptin and aldosterone levels was also observed in cardiac myofibroblasts of rats fed a high-fat diet. Here, the aldosterone antagonist eplerenone reduced the leptin-induced increase in protein levels of pro-fibrotic factors collagen I, TGFβ, connective tissue growth factor, and galectin-3, and decreased both total and mitochondrial ROS levels (Gutiérrez-Tenorio et al. 2017). In vitro experiments with human umbilical vein endothelial cells show that leptin causes chronic oxidative stress, which may enhance atherogenic processes and lead to the development of vascular disease (Bouloumié et al. 1999). Leptin can promote the proliferation and migration of vascular smooth muscle cells as well as the calcification of vascular cells, both of which contribute to the creation and progression of vascular lesions (Parhami et al. 2001).

Furthermore, it is widely assumed that leptin-mediated endothelial nitric oxide (NO) release promotes vasodilation and counteracts the suppressive impact of leptin-induced sympathoexcitatory activity.

Hyperleptinemia, on the other hand, resulted in lower NO bioavailability and attenuated NO-dependent vasodilation in individuals with obesity and T2DM, which contributes to vascular dysfunction (Kimura et al. 2000).

Hypertension

Obesity is commonly linked to an increased risk of hypertension, and there are robust associations between blood pressure and circulating leptin levels across a wide range of blood pressures (Haynes 2005). One possible explanation for these findings is that leptin resistance in obesity is selective for hypothalamic food intake regulation and leptin's ability to promote central sympathetic activity does not apply to the following peripheral effects including an increase in systemic pressor effect and a decrease in renal natriuresis, both of which contribute to hypertension (Rahmouni et al. 2012).

Research in which hypertension was produced by central overexpression of leptin and reversed by a leptin antagonist bolstered this idea. However, leptin antagonism did not affect high-fat diet-associated hypertension, calling the pathophysiological relevance of these findings into doubt (Tümer et al. 2007).

Notably, the positive relationship between leptin and hypertension has never been consistently observed, and age, gender, and race may all play a role. Furthermore, leptin treatment has no substantial immediate effect on blood pressure in healthy persons. Few investigations on hypertension in animal models have been conducted, yet both obese db/db mice and Zucker rats develop hypertension (Osmond et al. 2009). Obesity and hypertension are strongly linked, according to clinical and animal research (Rahmouni et al. 2005). The sympathetic cardiovascular effects of leptin may be one of the reasons connecting increased fat mass to hypertension. The sympathetic nervous system (SNS) overactivity, which is typical in the obese population, raises arterial pressure by producing peripheral vasoconstriction and enhancing renal tubular sodium reabsorption. An infusion of leptin produces sympathetic activity in several organs such as brown adipose tissue, kidney, and adrenal gland, according to experimental studies.

Leptin treatment raises plasma norepinephrine and epinephrine concentrations in a dose-dependent manner. Blood pressure rises as a result of sympathetic activation in response to leptin. Clinical research shows that leptin is also linked to mean blood pressure in obese people with essential hypertension. High leptin levels resulted in increased arterial pressure despite body weight decrease in transgenic mice with hyperleptinemia or after 12 days of exogenous leptin injection. Intracerebroventricular (ICV) treatment of leptin has been shown to elevate mean blood pressure slowly but steadily, as well as lumbar and renal sympathetic nerve activity (Dubinion, Da Silva, and Hall 2011).

Alpha-adrenergic or ganglionic inhibition prevented increased sympathetic activity. Obese persons with leptin insufficiency are also overweight yet have low blood pressure. This finding is similar to findings in leptin-deficient obese/obese mice: arterial pressures were lower, and leptin treatment increased systolic blood pressure. In addition, despite resistance to anorectic and weight-reducing effects in hyperleptinemia models such as diet-induced obesity (DIO) mice and agouti yellow obese mice, renal sympathetic activation of leptin was retained (Trevenzoli et al. 2010).

According to some research, leptin's sympathetic impact may be mediated via its activity in the hypothalamic arcuate nucleus (Harlan et al. 2011). These findings imply that leptin-induced sympathetic overactivity contributes to the development of hypertension in obese people.

Other factors, in addition to increased sympathetic activity, may contribute to the development of obesity-associated hypertension. Leptin, for example, boosted the production of several proinflammatory cytokines such as tumor necrosis factor (TNF)-α and interleukin (IL)-6 in endothelial cells. These are the causes of hypertension and atherosclerosis. Furthermore, leptin has been shown to stimulate the production of vasoconstrictor substances such as endothelin-1 (ET-1) and angiotensin II (AngII). However, other investigations have indicated that leptin has a direct vasodilating impact by stimulating the generation of nitric oxide (NO) in endothelial and smooth muscle cells (Rodríguez et al. 2007). Another experiment, however, revealed that there was no vasodilatory effect in conscious mice, and that blocking NO synthesis increased heart rate, renal vascular and glomerular response, but not significantly the suppressive response to leptin, with a negligible effect of leptin-stimulated NO production on blood pressure in vivo. It was discovered to play a role (Hou and Luo 2011).

Atherosclerosis

Leptin promotes and accelerates atherosclerosis through several processes, including intimal monocyte recruitment, macrophage transformation, vascular smooth muscle cell proliferation, and increased production of proatherogenic cytokines (Beltowski 2006). Experimental research indicates that leptin has a function in the etiology of atherosclerosis. Leptin-deficient ob/ob animals were resistant to atherosclerosis in vivo, whereas leptin directly exacerbated atherosclerosis in apolipoprotein E. Furthermore, leptin receptors have been found in human atherosclerosis, and clinical trials have demonstrated that plasma leptin concentrations are related to atherosclerosis in certain individuals (McMahon et al. 2011). An intriguing study discovered that leptin's proatherogenic effects on human monocytes are mediated by phosphoinositide 3 kinase and conventional protein kinase C signaling, and the actin cytoskeleton includes na+/H+ exchanger1 and NADPH oxidase (Konstantinidis et al. 2009).

These findings provide credence to the theory that leptin signaling promotes atherosclerosis. Hypertension, oxidative stress, endothelial dysfunction, inflammation, platelet aggregation, endothelial cell migration and proliferation, VSMC proliferation, migration, and calcification are all pro-atherogenic effects of leptin (Hou and Luo 2011).

Development of a Thrombus

Thrombus development is the leading cause of acute coronary events, particularly in obese people (Bodary 2007). Many investigations have demonstrated that leptin enhances platelet aggregation; nevertheless, this result may be concentration-dependent, with only high leptin levels being prothrombotic. Platelets from obese people are more responsive to leptin and exhibit more ADP-dependent aggregation than platelets from lean patients. Animal model studies also show that leptin has a prothrombotic impact; for example, OB/OB mice had decreased levels of thrombus formation, but this result is reversed with leptin administration. The mechanism of leptin-dependent platelet aggregation involves at least partially suppressed cGMP 3',5'-cyclic phosphodiesterase 3A, implying the possibility of pharmaceutical intervention (Elbatarny and Maurice 2005).

Furthermore, the pathophysiology of thrombosis implies that tissue factor (TF) plays a crucial role in the establishment of intracoronary thrombus. According to recent research, leptin stimulates the expression of TF and cellular adhesion molecules (CAM) on human coronary endothelial cells (HCAEC), which is controlled by eNOS generation of free oxygen radicals via nuclear factor (NF)-B activation (Cirillo et al. 2010). When taken as a whole. These findings support the notion that leptin has a unique relationship between obesity and cardiovascular events.

Conclusion

Leptin is a pleiotropic adipokine that has a variety of impacts on different cell types in the body. Leptin is the primary hormone that regulates energy balance and body fatness. Overall, it has been identified as an adipocyte-derived factor having pleiotropic effects on nutritional and metabolic status, immunological response and inflammation modulation, and cardiovascular function management. Its involvement in neuroendocrine signaling, homeostasis, and metabolism has also been extensively researched. Leptin has recently been recognized as a key immune modulator with a wide range of actions, the majority of which are pro-inflammatory.

Animal studies utilizing leptin- or LR-deficient rats demonstrate that cardiac failure is related to a metabolic transition from glucose metabolism to fatty acid oxidation, which promotes lipotoxicity, systemic inflammation, insulin resistance, and renin-angiotensin-aldosterone system activation. The intricacy of leptin receptor signaling, as well as the numerous variations of the receptor with distinct signaling capacities, allow for a wide range of mediated effects on various immune cells, which are sometimes located in the same tissues.

Because leptin regulates the cardiovascular system, it is crucial to create innovative techniques that target the influence of leptin on the cardiovascular system in normal and pathological settings. Future studies will be required to determine the specific role of leptin in various cardiac cell types such as cardiomyocytes, endothelial cells, and fibroblasts. As a result, transitioning from leptin- and Leptin-receptor-deficient rat models to human-based models will be critical for the development of novel treatment methods.

References

Abe, Yukiko, Koh Ono, Teruhisa Kawamura, Hiromichi Wada, Toru Kita, Akira Shimatsu, and Koji Hasegawa. 2007. "Leptin Induces Elongation of Cardiac Myocytes and Causes Eccentric Left Ventricular Dilatation with Compensation." *American Journal of Physiology - Heart and Circulatory Physiology* 292 (5): 2387–96. https://doi.org/10.1152/ajpheart.00579.2006.

Ahiante, Blessing O., Wayne Smith, Leandi Lammertyn, and Aletta E. Schutte. 2019. "Leptin and the Vasculature in Young Adults: The African-PREDICT Study." *European Journal of Clinical Investigation* 49 (1): 1–10. https://doi.org/10.1111/eci.13039.

Ahima, Rexford S., and Suzette Y. Osei. 2004. "Leptin Signaling." *Physiology and Behavior* 81 (2): 223–41. https://doi.org/10.1016/j.physbeh.2004.02.014.

Allison, Margaret B., and Martin G. Myers. 2014. "20 Years of Leptin: Connecting Leptin Signaling to Biological Function." *Journal of Endocrinology* 223 (1): T25–35. https://doi.org/10.1530/JOE-14-0404.

Amjad, Sofia, Mukhtiar Baig, Nida Zahid, Sundus Tariq, and Rehana Rehman. 2019. "Association between Leptin, Obesity, Hormonal Interplay and Male Infertility." *Andrologia* 51 (1): 1–7. https://doi.org/10.1111/and.13147.

Barouch, Lili A., Dan E. Berkowitz, Robert W. Harrison, Christopher P. O'Donnell, and Joshua M. Hare. 2003. "Disruption of Leptin Signaling Contributes to Cardiac Hypertrophy Independently of Body Weight in Mice." *Circulation* 108 (6): 754–59. https://doi.org/10.1161/01.CIR.0000083716.82622.FD.

Bełtowski, Jerzy. 2006. "Leptin and Atherosclerosis." *Atherosclerosis* 189 (1): 47–60. https://doi.org/10.1016/j.atherosclerosis.2006.03.003.

Bełtowski, Jerzy, Grazyna Wójcicka, and Anna Jamroz. 2003. "Leptin Decreases Plasma Paraoxonase 1 (PON1) Activity and Induces Oxidative Stress: The Possible Novel Mechanism for Proatherogenic Effect of Chronic Hyperleptinemia." *Atherosclerosis* 170 (1): 21–29. https://doi.org/10.1016/S0021-9150(03)00236-3.

Bobbert, Peter, Alexander Jenke, Thomas Bobbert, Uwe Kühl, Ursula Rauch, Dirk Lassner, Carmen Scheibenbogen, Wolfgang Poller, Heinz Peter Schultheiss, and Carsten Skurk. 2012. "High Leptin and Resistin Expression in Chronic Heart Failure: Adverse Outcome in Patients with Dilated and Inflammatory Cardiomyopathy." *European Journal of Heart Failure* 14 (11): 1265–75. https://doi.org/10.1093/eurjhf/hfs111.

Bodary, Peter F. 2007. "Links between Adipose Tissue and Thrombosis in the Mouse." *Arteriosclerosis, Thrombosis, and Vascular Biology* 27 (11): 2284–91. https://doi.org/10.1161/ATVBAHA.107.148221.

Boudina, Sihem, and E. Dale Abel. 2007. "Diabetic Cardiomyopathy Revisited." *Circulation* 115 (25): 3213–23. https://doi.org/10.1161/CIRCULATIONAHA.106.679597.

Bouloumié, Anne, Takeshi Marumo, Max Lafontan, and Rudi Busse. 1999. "Leptin Induces Oxidative Stress in Human Endothelial Cells." *The FASEB Journal* 13 (10): 1231–38. https://doi.org/10.1096/fasebj.13.10.1231.

Buchanan, Jonathan, Pradip K. Mazumder, Ping Hu, Gopa Chakrabarti, Matthew W. Roberts, Jeong Yun Ui, Robert C. Cooksey, Sheldon E. Litwin, and E. Dale Abel.

2005. "Reduced Cardiac Efficiency and Altered Substrate Metabolism Precedes the Onset of Hyperglycemia and Contractile Dysfunction in Two Mouse Models of Insulin Resistance and Obesity." *Endocrinology* 146 (12): 5341–49. https://doi.org/10.1210/en.2005-0938.

Chan, Jean L., Giuseppe Matarese, Greeshma K. Shetty, Patricia Raciti, Iosif Kelesidis, Daniela Aufiero, Veronica De Rosa, Francesco Perna, Silvia Fontana, and Christos S. Mantzoros. 2006. "Differential Regulation of Metabolic, Neuroendocrine, and Immune Function by Leptin in Humans." *Proceedings of the National Academy of Sciences of the United States of America* 103 (22): 8481–86. https://doi.org/10.1073/pnas.0505429103.

Cirillo, Plinio, Valeria Angri, Salvatore De Rosa, Gaetano Calì, Gianluca Petrillo, Fabio Maresca, Greta Luana D'Ascoli, Paola Maietta, Linda Brevetti, and Massimo Chiariello. 2010. "Pro-Atherothrombotic Effects of Leptin in Human Coronary Endothelial Cells." *Thrombosis and Haemostasis* 103 (5): 1065–75. https://doi.org/10.1160/TH09-06-0392.

Despres J. P. 2006. "Intra-Abdominal Obesity: An Untreated Risk Factor for Type 2 Diabetes and Cardiovascular Disease." *J. Endocrinol. Invest.* 29: 77–82.

Dong, F., X. Zhang, X. Yang, L. B. Esberg, H. Yang, Z. Zhang, B. Culver, and J. Ren. 2006. "Impaired Cardiac Contractile Function in Ventricular Myocytes from Leptin-Deficient Ob/Ob Obese Mice." *Journal of Endocrinology* 188 (1): 25–36. https://doi.org/10.1677/joe.1.06241.

Dornbush S., Aeddula N. R. 2023. *Physiology, Leptin.* StatPearls. Treasure Island (FL): StatPearls Publishing;

Dubinion, John H., Alexandre A. Da Silva, and John E. Hall. 2011. "Chronic Blood Pressure and Appetite Responses to Central Leptin Infusion in Rats Fed a High Fat Diet." *Journal of Hypertension* 29 (4): 758–62. https://doi.org/10.1097/HJH.0b013e3 28344280b.

Elbatarny, Hisham S., and Donald H. Maurice. 2005. "Leptin-Mediated Activation of Human Platelets: Involvement of a Leptin Receptor and Phosphodiesterase 3A-Containing Cellular Signaling Complex." *American Journal of Physiology - Endocrinology and Metabolism* 289 (4 52-4): 695–702. https://doi.org/10.1152/ajpendo.00125.2005.

Elif Arioglu Oral, MD., Vinaya Simha, M. D., Elaine Ruiz, N. P., Alexa Andewelt, B. S., Ahalya Premkumar, MD., Peter Snell, PhD., Anthony J. Wagner, PhD., Alex M. DePaoli, MD., Marc L. Reitman, MD., PhD., Simeon I. Taylor, MD., PhD., Phillip Gorden, MD. 2002. "Leptin-Replacement Therapy for Lipodystrophy." *N Engl J Med.* 346 (8): 570–78.

Farr, Olivia M., Gavirieli, Anna. 2017. "Leptin Applications in 2015: What Have We Learned about Leptin and Obesity." *Physiology & Behavior* 176 (12): 139–48. https://doi.org/10.1097/MED.0000000000000184.Leptin.

Funcke, Jan-Bernd, Julia von Schnurbein, Belinda Lennerz, Georgia Lahr, Klaus-Michael Debatin, Pamela Fischer-Posovszky, and Martin Wabitsch. 2014. "Monogenic Forms of Childhood Obesity Due to Mutations in the Leptin Gene." *Molecular and Cellular Pediatrics* 1 (1): 1–8. https://doi.org/10.1186/s40348-014-0003-1.

Gaal, Luc F. Van, Ilse L. Mertens, and Christophe E. De Block. 2006. "Mechanisms Linking Obesity with Cardiovascular Disease." *Nature* 444 (7121): 875–80. https://doi.org/10.1038/nature05487.

Golfman, Leonard S., Christopher R. Wilson, Saumya Sharma, Mathias Burgmaier, Martin E. Young, Patrick H. Guthrie, Melissa Van Arsdall, Julia V. Adrogue, Kathleen K. Brown, and Heinrich Taegtmeyer. 2005. "Activation of PPARγ Enhances Myocardial Glucose Oxidation and Improves Contractile Function in Isolated Working Hearts of ZDF Rats." *American Journal of Physiology - Endocrinology and Metabolism* 289 (2 52-2): 328–36. https://doi.org/10.1152/ajpendo.00055.2005.

Gong, Da Wei, Sheng Bi, Richard E. Pratley, and Bruce D. Weintraub. 1996. "Genomic Structure and Promoter Analysis of the Human Obese Gene." *Journal of Biological Chemistry* 271 (8): 3971–74. https://doi.org/10.1074/jbc.271.8.3971.

Gutiérrez-Tenorio, Josué, Gema Marín-Royo, Ernesto Martínez-Martínez, Rubén Martín, María Miana, Natalia López-Andrés, Raquel Jurado-López, Isabel Gallardo, María Luaces, José Alberto San Román, María González-Amor, Mercedes Salaices, María Luisa Nieto & Victoria Cachofeiro. 2017. "The Role of Oxidative Stress in the Crosstalk between Leptin and Mineralocorticoid Receptor in the Cardiac Fibrosis Associated with Obesity." *Scientific Reports* 7 (1): 1–9. https://doi.org/10.1038/s41598-017-17103-9.

Han, Xuefeng, Subat Turdi, Nan Hu, Rui Guo, Yingmei Zhang, and Jun Ren. 2012. "Influence of Long-Term Caloric Restriction on Myocardial and Cardiomyocyte Contractile Function and Autophagy in Mice." *Journal of Nutritional Biochemistry* 23 (12): 1592–99. https://doi.org/10.1016/j.jnutbio.2011.11.002.

Harlan, Shannon M., Donald A. Morgan, Khristofor Agassandian, Deng Fu Guo, Martin D. Cassell, Curt D. Sigmund, Allyn L. Mark, and Kamal Rahmouni. 2011. "Ablation of the Leptin Receptor in the Hypothalamic Arcuate Nucleus Abrogates Leptin-Induced Sympathetic Activation." *Circulation Research* 108 (7): 808–12. https://doi.org/10.1161/CIRCRESAHA.111.240226.

Haynes, William G. 2005. "Role of Leptin in Obesity-Related Hypertension." *Experimental Physiology* 90 (5): 683–88. https://doi.org/10.1113/expphysiol.2005.031237.

Hou, Ning, and Jian Dong Luo. 2011. "Leptin and Cardiovascular Diseases." *Clinical and Experimental Pharmacology and Physiology* 38 (12): 905–13. https://doi.org/10.1111/j.1440-1681.2011.05619.x.

Huby, Anne Cécile, Galina Antonova, Jake Groenendyk, Celso E. Gomez-Sanchez, Wendy B. Bollag, Jessica A. Filosa, and Eric J. Belin De Chantemèle. 2015. "Adipocyte-Derived Hormone Leptin Is a Direct Regulator of Aldosterone Secretion, Which Promotes Endothelial Dysfunction and Cardiac Fibrosis." *Circulation* 132 (22): 2134–45. https://doi.org/10.1161/CIRCULATIONAHA.115.018226.

Kiernan, Kaitlin, and Nancie J. MacIver. 2021. "The Role of the Adipokine Leptin in Immune Cell Function in Health and Disease." *Frontiers in Immunology* 11 (January): 1–11. https://doi.org/10.3389/fimmu.2020.622468.

Kimura, Keizo, Kazushi Tsuda, Akira Baba, Tetsuya Kawabe, Shin Ichi Boh-Oka, Masayo Ibata, Chizu Moriwaki, Takuzo Hano, and Ichiro Nishio. 2000. "Involvement of Nitric Oxide in Endothelium-Dependent Arterial Relaxation by Leptin." *Biochemical and*

Biophysical Research Communications 273 (2): 745–49. https://doi.org/10.1006/bbrc.2000.3005.

Konstantinides, Stavros, Katrin Schäfer, Jaap G. Neels, Claudia Dellas, and David J. Loskutoff. 2004. "Inhibition of Endogenous Leptin Protects Mice from Arterial and Venous Thrombosis." *Arteriosclerosis, Thrombosis, and Vascular Biology* 24 (11): 2196–2201. https://doi.org/10.1161/01.ATV.0000146531.79402.9a.

Konstantinidis, Diamantis, Konstantinos Paletas, George Koliakos, and Martha Kaloyianni. 2009. "Signaling Components Involved in Leptin-Induced Amplification of the Atherosclerosis-Related Properties of Human Monocytes." *Journal of Vascular Research* 46 (3): 199–208. https://doi.org/10.1159/000161234.

Korda, Mykhaylo, Ruslan Kubant, Stephen Patton, and Tadeusz Malinski. 2008. "Leptin-Induced Endothelial Dysfunction in Obesity." *American Journal of Physiology - Heart and Circulatory Physiology* 295 (4): 1514–21. https://doi.org/10.1152/ajpheart.00479.2008.

Liu, Jiankang, Kenneth R. Butler, Sarah G. Buxbaum, Jung Hye Sung, Brenda W. Campbell, and Herman A. Taylor. 2010. "Leptinemia and Its Association with Stroke and Coronary Heart Disease in the Jackson Heart Study." *Clinical Endocrinology* 72 (1): 32–37. https://doi.org/10.1111/j.1365-2265.2009.03627.x.

Mazumder, Pradip K., Brian T. O. Neill, Matthew W. Roberts, Jonathan Buchanan, Ui Jeong Yun, Robert C. Cooksey, Sihem Boudina, and E. Dale Abel. 2004. "Impaired Cardiac Efficiency and Increased Fatty Acid Oxidation in Insulin-Resistant Ob / Ob Mouse Hearts." *Diabetes* 53 (September): 2366–74. http://diabetes.diabetesjournals.org/content/diabetes/53/9/2366.full.pdf.

McMahon, Maureen, Brian J. Skaggs, Lori Sahakian, Jennifer Grossman, John FitzGerald, Nagesh Ragavendra, Christina Charles-Schoeman, Marissa Chernishof, Alan Gorn, Joseph L Witztum, Weng Kee Wong, Michael Weisman, Daniel J. Wallace, Antonio La Cava, Bevra H. Hahn. 2011. "High Plasma Leptin Levels Confer Increased Risk of Atherosclerosis in Women with Systemic Lupus Erythematosus, and Are Associated with Inflammatory Oxidised Lipids." *Annals of the Rheumatic Diseases* 70 (9): 1619–24. https://doi.org/10.1136/ard.2010.142737.

Nunziata, Adriana, Jan Bernd Funcke, Guntram Borck, Julia Von Schnurbein, Stephanie Brandt, Belinda Lennerz, Barbara Moepps, Peter Gierschik, Pamela Fischer-Posovszky, and Martin Wabitsch. 2019. "Functional and Phenotypic Characteristics of Human Leptin Receptor Mutations." *Journal of the Endocrine Society* 3 (1): 27–41. https://doi.org/10.1210/js.2018-00123.

Osmond, Jessica M., James D. Mintz, Brian Dalton, and David W. Stepp. 2009. "Obesity Increases Blood Pressure, Cerebral Vascular Remodeling, and Severity of Stroke in the Zucker Rat." *Hypertension* 53 (2): 381–86. https://doi.org/10.1161/HYPERTENSIONAHA.108.124149.

Ozata, M., I. C. Ozdemir, and J. Licinio. 1999. "Human Leptin Deficiency Caused by a Missense Mutation: Multiple Endocrine Defects, Decreased Sympathetic Tone, and Immune System Dysfunction Indicate New Targets for Leptin Action, Greater Central than Peripheral Resistance to the Effects of Leptin, and S." *J Clin Endocrinol Metab. 1999* 84 (10): 3686–95.

Parhami, Farhad, Yin Tintut, Alex Ballard, Alan M. Fogelman, and Linda L. Demer. 2001. "Leptin Enhances the Calcification of Vascular Cells Artery Wall as a Target of Leptin." *Circulation Research* 88 (9): 954–60. https://doi.org/10.1161/hh0901.090975.

Peelman, Frank, Lennart Zabeau, Kedar Moharana, Savvas N. Savvides, and Jan Tavernier. 2014. "Insights into Signaling Assemblies of the Leptin Receptor." *Journal of Endocrinology* 223 (1): T9–23. https://doi.org/10.1530/JOE-14-0264.

Peters, Triinu, Jochen Antel, Manuel Föcker, Simon Esber, Anke Hinney, Erik Schéle, Suzanne L. Dickson, Özgür Albayrak, and Johannes Hebebrand. 2018. "The Association of Serum Leptin Levels with Food Addiction Is Moderated by Weight Status in Adolescent Psychiatric Inpatients." *European Eating Disorders Review* 26 (6): 618–28. https://doi.org/10.1002/erv.2637.

Poetsch, Mareike S., Anna Strano, and Kaomei Guan. 2020. "Role of Leptin in Cardiovascular Diseases." *Frontiers in Endocrinology* 11 (June): 1–13. https://doi.org/10.3389/fendo.2020.00354.

Purdham, Daniel M., Min Xu Zou, Venkatesh Rajapurohitam, and Morris Karmazyn. 2004. "Rat Heart Is a Site of Leptin Production and Action." *American Journal of Physiology - Heart and Circulatory Physiology* 287 (6 56-6): 2877–84. https://doi.org/10.1152/ajpheart.00499.2004.

Racil, G., J. B. Coquart, W. Elmontassar, M. Haddad, R. Goebel, A. Chaouachi, M. Amri, and K. Chamari. 2016. "Greater Effects of High-Compared with Moderate-Intensity Interval Training on Cardio-Metabolic Variables, Blood Leptin Concentration and Ratings of Perceived Exertion in Obese Adolescent Females." *Biology of Sport* 33 (2): 145–52. https://doi.org/10.5604/20831862.1198633.

Rahmouni, Kamal, Marcelo L. G. Correia, William G. Haynes, and Allyn L. Mark. 2005. "Obesity-Associated Hypertension: New Insights into Mechanisms." *Hypertension* 45 (1): 9–14. https://doi.org/10.1161/01.HYP.0000151325.83008.b4.

Rahmouni, Kamal, Donald A Morgan, Gina M Morgan, Allyn L Mark, and William G Haynes. 2012. "Obesity Hypertension" 54 (July 2005).

Robertson, Lauren T., J. Humberto Treviño-Villarreal, Pedro Mejia, Yohann Grondin, Eylul Harputlugil, Christopher Hine, Dorathy Vargas, Hanqiao Zheng, C. Keith Ozaki, Bruce S. Kristal, Stephen J. Simpson, James R. Mitchell. 2015. "Protein and Calorie Restriction Contribute Additively to Protection from Renal Ischemia Reperfusion Injury Partly via Leptin Reduction in Male Mice." *Journal of Nutrition* 145 (8): 1717–27. https://doi.org/10.3945/jn.114.199380.

Rodríguez, Amaia, Ana Fortuño, Javier Gómez-Ambrosi, Guillermo Zalba, Javier Díez, and Gema Frühbeck. 2007. "The Inhibitory Effect of Leptin on Angiotensin II-Induced Vasoconstriction in Vascular Smooth Muscle Cells Is Mediated via a Nitric Oxide-Dependent Mechanism." *Endocrinology* 148 (1): 324–31. https://doi.org/10.1210/en.2006-0940.

Rogozina O. P., Bonorden M. J, Seppanen C. N., Grande J. P. and Cleary M. P. 2011. "Effect of Chronic and Intermittent Calorie Restriction on Serum Adiponectin and Leptin and Mammary Tumorigenesis." *Cancer Prev Res (Phila).* 4: 568–81. https://doi.org/10.1158/1940-6207.CAPR-10-0140.Effect.

Sadaf Farooqi, I., Giuseppe Matarese, Graham M. Lord, Julia M. Keogh, Elizabeth Lawrence, Chizo Agwu, Veronica Sanna, Susan A. Jebb, Francesco Perna, Silvia Fontana, Robert I. Lechler, Alex M. DePaoli, Stephen O'Rahilly. 2002. "Beneficial Effects of Leptin on Obesity, T Cell Hyporesponsiveness, and Neuroendocrine/Metabolic Dysfunction of Human Congenital Leptin Deficiency." *Journal of Clinical Investigation* 110 (8): 1093–1103. https://doi.org/10.1172/JCI200215693.

Sadaf Farooqi, I., and Stephen O'Rahilly. 2014. "20 Years of Leptin: Human Disorders of Leptin Action." *Journal of Endocrinology* 223 (1): T63–70. https://doi.org/10.1530/JOE-14-0480.

Sharma, Saumya, Julia V. Adrogue, Leonard Golfman, Ivan Uray, John Lemm, Keith Youker, George P. Noon, O. H. Frazier, and Heinrich Taegtmeyer. 2004. "Intramyocardial Lipid Accumulation in the Failing Human Heart Resembles the Lipotoxic Rat Heart." *The FASEB Journal* 18 (14): 1692–1700. https://doi.org/10.1096/fj.04-2263com.

Shinmura, Ken, Kayoko Tamaki, Motoaki Sano, Mitsushige Murata, Hiroyuki Yamakawa, Hideyuki Ishida, and Keiichi Fukuda. 2011. "Impact of Long-Term Caloric Restriction on Cardiac Senescence: Caloric Restriction Ameliorates Cardiac Diastolic Dysfunction Associated with Aging." *Journal of Molecular and Cellular Cardiology* 50 (1): 117–27. https://doi.org/10.1016/j.yjmcc.2010.10.018.

Sinha, Madhur K, Jeppe Sturis, Joanna Ohannesian, Susan Magosin, F Caro, Thomas Stephens, Mark L Heiman, and Kenneth S Polonsky. 1996. "Ultradian Oscillations of Leptin Secretion in Humans between Midnight and Early Morning Hours and Lowest around Noon to Mid-Afternoon. In " *Biochemical and Biophysical Research Communications* 738: 733–38.

Trevenzoli, I. H., C. R. Pinheiro, E. P. S. Conceição, E. Oliveira, M. C. F. Passos, P. C. Lisboa, and E. G. Moura. 2010. "Programming of Rat Adrenal Medulla by Neonatal Hyperleptinemia: Adrenal Morphology, Catecholamine Secretion, and Leptin Signaling Pathway." *American Journal of Physiology - Endocrinology and Metabolism* 298 (5): 941–49. https://doi.org/10.1152/ajpendo.00734.2009.

Tümer, Nihal, Benedek Erdös, Michael Matheny, Idan Cudykier, and Philip J. Scarpace. 2007. "Leptin Antagonist Reverses Hypertension Caused by Leptin Overexpression, but Fails to Normalize Obesity-Related Hypertension." *Journal of Hypertension* 25 (12): 2471–78. https://doi.org/10.1097/HJH.0b013e3282e9a9fd.

Wallace, A. Michael, Alex D. McMahon, Chris J. Packard, Anne Kelly, James Shepherd, Allan Gaw, and Naveed Sattar. 2001. "Plasma Leptin and the Risk of Cardiovascular Disease in the West of Scotland Coronary Prevention Study (WOSCOPS)." *Circulation* 104 (25): 3052–56. https://doi.org/10.1161/hc5001.101061.

Wasim, Muhammad, Fazli Rabbi Awan, Syeda Sadia Najam, Abdul Rehman Khan, and Haq Nawaz Khan. 2016. "Role of Leptin Deficiency, Inefficiency, and Leptin Receptors in Obesity." *Biochemical Genetics* 54 (5): 565–72. https://doi.org/10.1007/s10528-016-9751-z.

Welsh, Paul, Heather M. Murray, Brendan M. Buckley, Anton J. M. De Craen, Ian Ford, J. Wouter Jukema, Peter W. Macfarlane, Chris J. Packard, David J. Stott, Rudi G. J. Westendorp, James Shepherd, Naveed Sattar. 2009. "Leptin Predicts Diabetes but Not

Cardiovascular Disease: Results from a Large Prospective Study in an Elderly Population." *Diabetes Care* 32 (2): 308–10. https://doi.org/10.2337/dc08-1458.

"WHO. World Health Statistics Overview 2019: Monitoring Health for the SDGs, Sustainable Development Goals. Geneva: World Health Organization; (2019) (WHO/DAD/2019.1). Licence: CC BY-NC-SA 3.0 IGO. [Google Scholar]." n.d.

Ye, Feng, Aung Than, Yanying Zhao, Kian Hong Goh, and Peng Chen. 2010. "Vesicular Storage, Vesicle Trafficking, and Secretion of Leptin and Resistin: The Similarities, Differences, and Interplays." *Journal of Endocrinology* 206 (1): 27–36. https://doi.org/10.1677/JOE-10-0090.

Yue, Patrick, Takayasu Arai, Masahiro Terashima, Ahmad Y. Sheikh, Feng Cao, David Charo, Grant Hoyt, Robert C. Robbins, Euan A. Ashley, Joseph Wu, Phillip C. Yang and Philip S. Tsao. 2007. "Magnetic Resonance Imaging of Progressive Cardiomyopathic Changes in the Db/Db Mouse." *American Journal of Physiology - Heart and Circulatory Physiology* 292 (5): 2106–18. https://doi.org/10.1152/ajpheart.00856.2006.

Zhao, Shangang, Christine M. Kusminski, Joel K. Elmquist, and Philipp E. Scherer. 2020. "Leptin: Less Is More." *Diabetes* 69 (5): 823–29. https://doi.org/10.2337/dbi19-0018.

Zhao, Shangang, Christine M. Kusminski, and Philipp E. Scherer. 2021. "Adiponectin, Leptin and Cardiovascular Disorders." *Circulation Research* 128 (1): 136–49. https://doi.org/10.1161/CIRCRESAHA.120.314458.

Zhao, Shangang, Na Li, Yi Zhu, Leon Straub, Zhuzhen Zhang, May Yun Wang, Qingzhang Zhu, Christine M. Kusminski, Joel K. Elmquist, and Philipp E. Scherer. 2020. "Partial Leptin Deficiency Confers Resistance to Diet-Induced Obesity in Mice." *Molecular Metabolism* 37 (April): 1–12. https://doi.org/10.1016/j.molmet.2020.100995.

Chapter 4

Leptin in Reproductive Health and Disease

D. G. Kishor Kumar[1]
Ayushi Vaidhya[1]
C. L. Madhu[1]
Manjit Panigrahi[2]
T. U. Singh[1]
Dinesh Kumar[1]
and Subhashree Parida[1,*]

[1]Division of Pharmacology and Toxicology, ICAR-Indian Veterinary Research Institute, Izatnagar, Bareilly, Uttar Pradesh, India
[2]Division of Animal Genetics and Breeding, ICAR-Indian Veterinary Research Institute, Izatnagar, Bareilly, Uttar Pradesh, India

Abstract

Leptin, besides its role in regulating body weight, also plays a significant part in various physiological functions, including reproduction. It acts as a central player in the intricate signaling pathways of the hypothalamic-pituitary-gonadal axis, influencing multiple regions. Leptin receptors are found in the arcuate and ventromedial nucleus of the hypothalamus and the adenohypophysis, suggesting that leptin can impact the brain and/or anterior pituitary to modulate the secretion of GnRH and gonadotropins. Particularly during puberty, leptin can act as a metabolic gate in both males and females.

---

*Corresponding Author's Emails: subhaparida1210@gmail.com, subhashree.parida@icar.gov.in.

In: Leptin and its Role in Health and Disease
Editor: Stephen E. Bradley
ISBN: 979-8-89113-274-0
© 2024 Nova Science Publishers, Inc.

Furthermore, leptin receptors have been identified in female reproductive organs such as the ovary, uterus, placenta, blastocyst, fetal tissues, and mammary epithelial cells. This suggests that leptin may regulate various functions in these organs, including ovarian function, oocyte maturation, embryo development, implantation, placentation, pregnancy, fetal growth, and development, as well as lactation. During pregnancy, the concentration of leptin in the bloodstream significantly increases but decreases after birth, indicating its crucial role during gestation. By suppressing spontaneous and oxytocin-induced myometrial contractions, leptin may be involved in complications related to fetal delivery, particularly in obese females.

Disruptions in metabolic pathways involving leptin could potentially contribute to conditions like pre-eclampsia, leading to compromised intrauterine growth and abnormal birth weight and body composition in offspring. Obese females with elevated leptin levels are at a higher risk of experiencing adverse pregnancy outcomes, including gestational diabetes and hypertensive disorders of pregnancy. In males, leptin at physiological levels may aid in spermatogenesis, while higher levels of serum leptin have been negatively associated with low androgen levels, low sperm count, testicular oxidative stress, and increased morphological abnormalities in sperm among obese men. Leptin can traverse the blood-testes barrier, potentially impairing sperm development and the components of the blood-testis barrier in mice. Even slight variations in leptin levels can lead to infertility in both sexes.

The objective of this book chapter is to shed light on the reproductive functions of leptin and its role in altered reproductive physiology.

Introduction

"Nature has invented reproduction as a mechanism for life to move forward. As a life force that passes right through us and makes us a link in the evolution of life."

Louie Schwartzberg

Reproduction is a crucial aspect of species survival and confers an evolutionary advantage on Earth. On an individual level, the arrival of a child brings profound purpose to a person's life. The profound significance of reproduction becomes evident when considering the emotional pain and anguish experienced by couples struggling with infertility. While the primary components of reproduction involve the ovum, sperm, and uterus, numerous hidden factors contribute to the intricate process. Among these factors, leptin, a multifunctional hormone-cum-cytokine, plays a vital role. Deletion or dysfunction of leptin has been observed to result in infertility in both humans and mice. Understanding the role of leptin as one of the many essential ingredients in successful reproduction enhances our comprehension of the complex mechanisms involved and may offer potential avenues for addressing reproductive challenges.

Leptin, known as an adipokine due to its secretion primarily from adipose tissue, emerged as the most recent addition to the realm of known hormones. Its discovery took place in the 1990s, yet the gene responsible for producing this protein had been known to the scientific community as early as the 1950s. Notably, the deletion of both alleles of this gene led to obesity in mice, earning it the name "Ob gene." Additionally, these mice were found to be infertile, further highlighting the gene's significance. Despite the gene's identification, its function and true nature remained enigmatic. In a series of elegant experiments involving parabiosis in mice, the Coleman group in the 1960s uncovered the role of the protein encoded by the Ob gene in appetite suppression (Hummel et al., 1966; Coleman, 1978). Subsequently, the Friedman group conducted positional cloning of the Ob gene in the early 1990s, leading to the identification of the hormone and its official naming as leptin (Zhang et al., 1994).

The primary role of leptin, hence earning its name from the Greek word 'leptos' meaning thin, is to prevent obesity in mice. This hormone is often referred to as the "leaning hormone." Leptin receptors were initially characterized in db/db mice, a strain with diabetes that exhibited a strikingly similar phenotype to the Ob/Ob mice (Bates and Myers, 2003). Interestingly, db/db mice and patients with type II diabetes share a common feature: they develop leptin resistance despite having elevated levels of circulating leptin, paralleling the insulin resistance observed in individuals with elevated plasma insulin.

Apart from adipose tissue, leptin is also released in fewer amounts by the placenta, bone marrow, mammary epithelium, skeletal muscle, pituitary, hypothalamus, and stomach (Masuzaki et al., 1997; Bado et al., 1998; Morash et al., 1999; Ozata et al., 1999; Ahima and Flier, 2000). In addition to the regulation of food intake and body weight, leptin plays a key role in angiogenesis, hematopoiesis, lipid and carbohydrate metabolism and affects the functions of reproductive, cardiovascular, and immune systems (Wauters et al., 2000; Caprio et al., 2001; Hynes and Jones, 2001). Leptin represents an interesting target for studying the molecular interactions between the immune, neuronal, digestive and reproductive systems (Chehab et al., 1997). Its functions are pleiotropic, as indicated by its production in various tissues, implicated in a variety of cellular processes, including immune cell function. Leptin is structurally related to the long-chain helical cytokine family, which includes growth hormone, ciliary neurotrophic factor (CNTF), oncostatin-M (OSM), cardiotrophin-1 (CT-1), leukemia inhibitory factor (LIF) as well as interleukins (IL) such as IL-6, IL-2, IL-11 and IL-12 (Madej et al., 1995; Kline et al., 1997; Zhang et al., 1997; Frühbeck et al., 1998; Prolo et al., 1998; Frühbeck, 2006). Leptin produces most of its biological functions via the JAK/STAT pathway (Frühbeck, 2006).

Leptin Receptors

The leptin receptor family consists of single-membrane spanning receptors hallmarked by the presence of one or more cytokine receptor homology (CRH) domains. All receptors are devoid of intrinsic kinase activity and use JAK kinases for intracellular signaling. Six leptin receptor isoforms (ObRa-f) are generated by alternative splicing of the lepr gene (aka diabetes/db gene) (Münzberg and Morrison, 2015). ObRs are categorized into three groups: secreted, short, and long isoforms. ObRe is the secreted and the smallest isoform, contains neither the cytoplasmic nor the transmembrane domains but only the extracellular domains that can bind to circulating leptin and is either produced from alternatively spliced messenger RNA species (in the mouse) or from proteolytic cleavage of the membrane-bound form (in human) (Maamra et al., 2001; Bates and Myers, 2004; Münzberg et al., 2005). The short forms of ObRs are ObRa, ObRc, ObRd, and ObRf in rodents, whereas ObRb is classified as the long form. Leptin binds to both the short and long form receptors with the same affinity. However, only the long form has the capacity of strong leptin signaling as compared to others and initiates the necessary intracellular responses (Baumann et al., 1996; Rosenblum et al., 1996). The short and long forms of the ObRs are distinguished by the size of their intracellular domain and the presence of JAK/STAT binding sites. The long form (ObRb) has a 304 residue-large intracellular domain and has many JAK and STAT binding sites, whereas the short form (ObRa) comprises a small intracellular domain consisting of 34 residues and only one well-known JAK binding domain (Kelesidis et al., 2010). The shorter isoforms, ObRa, ObRc, ObRd, and ObRf have been identified in multiple species and possess truncated cytoplasmic domains with reduced signaling transduction capability. The short forms of ObR cannot mediate leptin-induced changes in energy homeostasis (Murakami et al., 1997).

Leptin receptor expression has been observed in various species, indicating its significance in reproductive processes. In wild animals such as Japanese black bears, leptin receptors have been found in the uterus (Nakamura et al., 2009). In nonpregnant heifers, leptin receptor mRNA is expressed throughout the estrus cycle, with the highest expression during the luteal phase (Sosa et al., 2010). In humans, leptin receptor expression in the endometrium has been linked to endometriosis (Kitawaki et al., 2000). Both mRNA and protein of the leptin receptor have been detected in the endometrial glands and mesenchyma (Liu et al., 2003). Similar findings have been reported in pigs, with ObRb mRNA expression observed in the uterus (Lin et al., 2000) and leptin receptor protein expression in the placenta (Ashworth et al., 2000).

Leptin receptor expression has also been investigated in mice, humans, and rabbits during early pregnancy (Señarís et al., 1997; Hoggard et al., 1997; González et al., 2000; Kawamura et al., 2003, Gonzalez and Leavis, 2003). In these species, ObRb mRNA and protein have been detected in the endometrium, placental trophoblastic cells, and myometrium. Porcine studies have identified short forms of leptin receptor expression in the endometrium and myometrium during the luteal phase and early pregnancy, with ObRb expression peaking on days 14-16 of the cycle (Bogacka et al., 2006, Smolinska et al., 2007). Additionally, leptin receptors have been found in the myometrium of mice during early pregnancy (Harrod et al., 2011). In dogs, leptin receptors are expressed in both the myometrial and endometrial layers of the uterus, as well as in the placenta during pregnancy (Balogh et al., 2015).

Furthermore, alterations in leptin receptor expression have been observed in certain conditions. For instance, in a rat model of gestational hypertension, placental expression of leptin receptors was increased (Anderson et al., 2005). These findings highlight the involvement of leptin receptors in reproductive physiology and suggest their potential role in reproductive disorders and pregnancy-related complications.

Leptin Signaling

Leptin receptors belong to the class I cytokine receptor family which is known to act through JAKs (Janus kinases) and STATs (signal transducers and activators of transcription). In the hypothalamus region, leptin specifically activates the STAT3 pathway (Håkansson-Ovesjö et al., 2000). There are various signaling pathways known to mediate the actions of leptin and include JAK-STAT signaling, PI3K-Akt-FoxO1 signaling, SHP2-ERK signaling, AMPK signaling, and mTOR-S6K signaling. In contrast, signaling molecules/pathways mitigating leptin actions in hypothalamic neurons have been extensively studied in an effort to overcome leptin resistance observed in obesity. These include SOCS3, tyrosine phosphatase PTP1B, and inflammatory signaling pathways such as IKK-NFκB signaling, JNK signaling, and ER stress–mitochondrial signaling (Kwon et al., 2016). Missense mutations in the leptin receptor have been reported and are known to disrupt ObR signaling (Kimber et al., 2008). Defects in leptin signaling can cause severe obesity (Nanjappa et al., 2011).

Leptin in Female Reproduction

Leptin is implicated in the control of female reproductive functions including the physiology of puberty, regulation of functions of the ovary, maturation of the oocyte, ovulation, development of embryo, implantation, and placentation (Cervero et al., 2005; Dos Santos et al., 2012). Leptin plays a central role in reproduction by participating in the composite interplay of signaling pathways at several regions of the hypothalamic-pituitary-gonadal axis (Pérez-Pérez et al., 2015).

Leptin in the Physiology of Puberty

The onset of puberty is influenced by various factors, including the individual's nutritional condition, as many aspects of reproductive physiology require significant energy expenditure. Epidemiological studies in humans have suggested that an adequate amount of body fat is necessary for appropriate sexual maturation to occur. The onset of puberty is regulated by the interaction of two physiological processes: adrenarche and gonadarche. Adrenarche involves the secretion of steroid hormones (such as androstenedione, dehydroepiandrosterone, and cortisol), as well as insulin-like growth factor and growth hormone, by the adrenal cortex. These hormones contribute to the pubertal growth spurt, body odor, and skeletal maturation. Gonadarche, on the other hand, involves the activation of the hypothalamic-pituitary-gonadal (HPG) axis. Various hormones including leptin have been identified to participate in the activation of the HPG axis. Leptin's role in gonadarche is more profound compared to that in adrenache (Nieuwenhuis et al., 2020). During gonadarche, leptin has the ability to stimulate the secretion of kisspeptin, a key regulator of reproductive function which in turn activates the hypothalamic-pituitary-gonadal (HPG) axis. This activation leads to increased expression of estrogen and androstenedione in the ovaries. In a reciprocal manner, estrogen generated from HPG axis activation stimulates the expression of the Ob gene in white adipose tissue, resulting in the synthesis and release of leptin. Hence, elevated levels of leptin play a role in promoting the onset of puberty in girls by stimulating the secretion of kisspeptin, while estrogen additionally stimulates the secretion of leptin.

Since its identification as a hormone originating from adipocytes in 1994, leptin has been widely acknowledged as a potential mediator between energy stores (adiposity) and the onset of puberty. External administration of leptin accelerated puberty in normal female mice and sexual maturation in leptin-deficient (ob/ob) mice (Ahima et al., 1997; Chehab et al., 1997) and thus leptin may be a permissive factor or a metabolic trigger in the attainment of puberty (Ahima et al., 1997; Chehab et al., 1997; Cheung et al., 1997; Demerath et al., 1999). The circulating leptin concentrations are generally higher in females than in males (Shimizu et al., 1997; Blum, 1997). Attainment of certain body weight along with age is critical for the onset of puberty and leptin could act as a metabolic gate, especially at the time of puberty (Barb and Kraeling, 2004). Serum leptin concentration was higher during puberty in mice (Chehab et al., 1997), heifers (Garcia et al., 2002), and pigs (Qian et al., 1999). The location of the ObRb receptor varies with species, but ObRb mRNA was reported to be localized in the arcuate and the ventromedial nucleus of the hypothalamus and adenohypophysis of mice (Tartaglia et al., 1995), rats (Zamorano et al., 1997), ewes (Dyer et al., 1997) and pigs (Lin et al., 2001). Thus, leptin can act at the level of the brain and/or anterior pituitary to modulate gonadotropin secretion. It has been also reported that leptin directly acts on arcuate neurons that produce gonadotropin-releasing hormone (GnRH) (Sullivan and Meonter, 2004). By inhibiting NPY and stimulating proopiomelanocortin POMC activity, leptin regulates GnRH/ LH secretion in primates (Kaynard et al., 1990), rodents (Kalra, 1993) and farm animals such as cows (Thomas et al., 1999), ewes (Morrison et al., 2003) and pigs (Barb, 1999). Treatment with leptin enhanced sexual maturation in both restricted diet-fed and ad lib diet-fed animals (Barash et al., 1996; Ahima et al., 1997).

Leptin in Ovarian Function

Leptin is also involved in the direct regulation of ovarian function. Leptin is found in follicular fluid with levels in accordance with those reported in serum (Cioffi et al., 1997). ObRs have been found in interstitial, theca, and granulosa cells of the ovary in humans (Cioffi et al., 1997; Karlsson et al., 1997). Leptin plays a significant role in the maturation of ovarian follicles and oocytes (Childs et al., 2021). It has been observed that all ovarian follicular cells possess leptin receptors, and physiological levels of leptin stimulate the maturation of granulosa cells, theca cells, and oocytes. Numerous studies have demonstrated the stimulatory effect of leptin on these target cells. In conjunction with growth factors like insulin-like growth factor-1 (IGF-1), growth hormone (GH), and follicle-stimulating hormone (FSH), physiological levels of leptin promote the development of follicles up to the antral stage. Furthermore, in partnership with luteinizing hormone (LH), leptin facilitates ovulation and oocyte maturation. As estradiol levels rise from the granulosa cells of the follicles, leptin levels also increase. Leptin, along with LH and growth factors, acts synergistically to promote oocyte meiosis and the formation of the polar body.

Leptin in Pregnancy

Embryo Implantation

The implantation of the embryo is a pivotal and essential step in pregnancy. During this process, the blastocyst establishes intimate attachment to the surface of the endometrium, leading to the formation of the placenta. Implantation is facilitated by a complex interplay of signaling events that are crucial for the successful establishment of pregnancy. Various mediators, including hormones, have been proposed to participate in this initial interaction between the fetus and the mother. Both leptin and ObRs are reported to be expressed in both the luminal and glandular tissues of the endometrial layer of the uterus throughout the menstrual cycle (Kitawaki et al., 2000; Cervero et al., 2005; Craig et al., 2005). The lower leptin receptor levels reported in the early proliferative phase that is followed by a gradual rise that peaks during the early secretory phase of the cycle may suggest that leptin receptor may be regulated by ovarian steroids and has a physiological role in the implantation of embryo (González et al., 2000). Leptin has been found to play a role in inducing blastocyst adhesion by upregulating the expression of αv and β3 integrin in endometrial epithelial cells. Integrins are cell surface proteins that are involved in cell adhesion and communication with the extracellular matrix. The αvβ3 integrin, in particular, has been shown to be important for the interaction between the blastocyst and the endometrium during implantation. Leptin increases the level of expression of matrix metalloproteinases (MMP) like MMP-2 and MMP-9 in cytotrophoblasts which are required during trophoblast invasion (Bischof et al., 2000; Castellucci, 2000; Fontana et al., 2010), suggesting the role of leptin in implantation. Leptin has been implicated in inducing implantation-related inflammation, which can stimulate the production of interleukin 6 (IL-6) and chemokines in endometrial epithelial cells (EECs) and endometrial stromal cells (ESCs). Leptin has been associated with the remodeling of the endometrial epithelium by promoting cellular proliferation and enhancing apoptosis induced by Fas ligand in endometrial epithelial cells (EECs). Leptin also contributes to the regenerative processes that occur in the endometrial epithelium after the successful implantation of the embryo. It is thought to participate in the repair and restoration of the endometrial lining, which undergoes changes during implantation and subsequent pregnancy. In contrary, elevated levels of leptin can interfere with the normal differentiation and transformation of endometrial stromal cells into decidual cells. This interference disrupts the formation of the decidua, which is crucial for the successful implantation and maintenance of pregnancy.

Placental Function

Leptin and its receptors are shown to be localized in the syncytiotrophoblast of the human placenta (Challier et al., 2003) indicating leptin may be involved in placental function and a regulator of endocrine functions of the placenta (Coya et al., 2006). The leptin derived from the human placenta is similar to the one derived from fat in size, charge, and immunoreactivity (Lappas et al., 2005), however, the expression of the leptin gene is modulated differently in placental tissue when compared to fat tissue as it possesses a placental leptin enhancer region which is a specific upstream enhancer (Ebihara et al., 1997).

All six isoforms of the leptin receptor have been reported from the human placenta (Challier et al., 2003). It is well known that leptin stimulates the JAK-STAT pathway which is proposed to be involved in trophoblast invasiveness

(Corvinus et al., 2003). As discussed in previous sections, leptin mediates the signal transduction pathways such as MAPK which mediates a proliferative response, and PI3K which is involved in the invasiveness of human trophoblast (Pollheimer and Knöfler, 2005; Pérez-Pérez et al., 2008). Leptin produced from the placenta triggers human chorionic gonadotropin (hCG) synthesis in trophoblast cells and enhances the production of metalloproteinases (MMP-2 and MMP-9) and extracellular matrix proteins that play an important role in extracellular matrix remodeling (Fontana et al., 2010). Hence, through JAK-STAT signaling, MAPK signaling, and PI3K signaling pathways (Martín-Romero and Sánchez-Margalet, 2001; Sánchez-Margalet and Martín-Romero, 2001; Pérez-Pérez et al., 2009; Pérez-Pérez et al., 2010), leptin stimulates growth, proliferation, and survival of trophoblastic cells (Pérez-Pérez et al., 2008). The involvement of Sam68, an RNA-binding protein that mediates the growth-enhancing effect of leptin, has been reported in trophoblastic cells (Sánchez-Jiménez et al., 2011; Sánchez-Jiménez et al., 2011a).

Furthermore, leptin influences placental hormone production. It has been shown to stimulate the synthesis and secretion of human chorionic gonadotropin (hCG) by trophoblast cells (Cameo et al., 2003). hCG is essential for the maintenance of pregnancy and is involved in various processes such as implantation and maternal immune tolerance towards the fetus. Leptin also modulates placental nutrient transport. It regulates the expression and activity of nutrient transporters in the placenta, including glucose transporters and amino acid transporters (Pérez-Pérez et al., 2020). This ensures an adequate supply of nutrients to support fetal growth and development. Additionally, leptin is implicated in placental angiogenesis and vascularization (Cao et al., 2001). It promotes the formation of new blood vessels in the placenta through the activation of angiogenic factors. This is crucial for adequate blood supply to the developing fetus and efficient exchange of oxygen and nutrients between the mother and the fetus. Overall, leptin plays a multifaceted role in placental function, including regulating trophoblast cell growth, hormone production, nutrient transport, and angiogenesis.

Uterine Contractions

The expression of leptin receptor isoform proteins in tissues such as the endometrium, placenta, blastocyst, fetal tissues, and mammary epithelial cells suggests that leptin could play a key part in pregnancy, growth, and development of the fetus and during lactation (Pérez-Pérez et al., 2015). Leptin suppresses both spontaneous and oxytocin-induced myometrial contractions (Moynihan et al., 2006; Mumtaz et al., 2015). The serum concentration of leptin significantly increases during pregnancy and decreases after birth, suggesting an important role during gestation (Briana and Malamitsi-Puchner, 2009). In a mouse model of pregnancy, the leptin-induced uterine response was receptor-dependent and was mediated by the JAK-STAT pathway. Short forms of leptin receptor mRNA and protein were reported from the uterus of late pregnant mice and, were located in the luminal epithelium and myometrial layers of the endometrium. The relaxant response was mediated by both NO and cGMP induced by leptin (Srinivasan et al., 2021). However, it is worth noting that conflicting results and observations have been reported in different studies, and the role of leptin in uterine contractions is still not fully understood. Notably, conditional knockout of the leptin receptor in the female reproductive tract reduced fertility due to parturition defects in mice, indicating an essential role of leptin in the induction of normal labor (Pennington et al., 2022).

Leptin in Reproductive Diseases

As far as female hormonology is concerned, the association between reproduction and metabolism has long been an issue of debate. Amino acids, insulin, and low-molecular-weight IGF-Binding Protein-1 (IGFBP-1) have been identified as beneficial signals in changes in body fat variation and BMI, although these changes have been linked to leptin levels (Goumenou et al., 2003). In addition to controlling obesity, leptin is crucial for regulating endocrine, reproductive, and immunological health by reducing calorie intake and increasing calorie expenditure. Thus, leptin plays a crucial role in many biological functions and numerous pathologies are linked to unusually elevated or decreased leptin levels (Cai et al., 2009). As discussed earlier, female reproduction and neuroendocrine function are mainly regulated by leptin, so it can be used as a therapy for infertility, eating disorders, and exercise-induced bone loss. Leptin acts at a very narrow concentration range and slight variations in leptin levels may lead to infertility in both sexes.

Aberrant metabolic pathways involving leptin may play a decisive role in pre-eclampsia and give rise to compromised intrauterine growth conditions and aberrant birth weight and body composition of offspring (Gurugubelli Krishna and Vishnu Bhat, 2018; de Knegt et al., 2021). Obese females with elevated leptin levels are likely to experience adverse pregnancy outcomes such as gestational diabetes and hypertensive disorders of pregnancy (Plowden et al., 2020). Higher leptin levels as seen in obese women can be detrimental to embryonic development (Broughton and Moley, 2017). Kinks in the leptin signaling pathway has been suggested as one of the probable causes of idiopathic recurrent pregnancy losses as indicated by a rise in serum leptin concentrations in recurrent pregnancy losses in women (Zidan et al., 2015; Serazin et al., 2018). The clinical onset of pre-eclampsia correlates with higher serum leptin levels and thus, leptin could be used as one of the biomarkers to predict the onset or diagnosis of pre-eclampsia (Anim-Nyame et al., 2000; de Knegt et al., 2021).

Higher leptin levels in ovaries reduce the production of estradiol and attenuate the development of dominant follicles and maturation of the oocyte, thus predisposing to anovulation. In case of the polycystic ovarian syndrome and obesity where there are metabolic disturbances or excess energy stores, leptin has a suppressive effect on the gonads (Pérez-Pérez et al., 2015). Hyperleptinemia (50–200 ng/ml) has been characterised by suppression of oocyte maturation and reduced follicular count. Leptin is also speculated to play a key role in ovulation as surge in leptin levels occurs at the same time as the LH surge prior to ovulation. Therefore, hyperleptinemia may also contribute to infertility by attenuating ovulation (Brannian and Hansen, 2002; Broughton and Moley, 2017; Baig et al., 2019; Childs et al., 2021).

Polycystic Ovarian Syndrome

Polycystic ovarian syndrome (PCOS) is characterized by chronic oligoovulation or anovulation, hyperandrogenism, and polycystic ovaries and is one of the most prevalent endocrine disorders affecting 5–10% of reproductive-age women. It is also the most common cause of anovulatory infertility (Azziz et al., 2004; Chen et al., 2013; Jaiswar and Priyadarshini, 2021). Clinical observations seen in PCOS are often associated with hyperleptinemia and it implies that leptin could take part in etiopathogenesis of the disease (Vázquez et al., 2015; Behboudi-Gandevani et al., 2017; Jaiswar and Priyadarshini, 2021). Leptin acts centrally to modulate the GnRH/gonadotropin axis, whose secretory activity is altered in PCOS (Löffler et al., 2001). Leptin also acts directly at the level of ovary, where it has been shown to be expressed in the ovaries of PCOS patients, and where direct leptin effects may help in follicular maturation and ovulation. Leptin may also be a factor in the insulin resistance and hyperandrogenism that are seen in the majority of PCOS patients (Escobar-Morreale and San Millán, 2007). It has been reported that the elevated concentrations of LH observed in women with PCOS were also associated with increased leptin levels (Chen et al., 2013) and nearly half of these women were obese, hence hyperleptinemia could be a common association in PCOS. Several other works have reported that PCOS is characterized by elevated levels of leptin (Brzechffa et al., 1996; Sharif and Rizk, 2015). Leptin may also be responsible for the pro-inflammatory and hyperandrogenic state noticed in PCOS (Escobar-Morreale and San Millán, 2007). Hypothalamic Kiss1 neurons are likely to be suppressed by long-term hyperleptinemia, which may also be a factor in some phenotypic PCOS symptoms such as ovulatory abnormalities (Quennell et al., 2011; Vázquez et al., 2015).

Recurrent Miscarriage

Recurrent miscarriage refers to the unfortunate occurrence of three or more consecutive pregnancy losses, whether or not there have been any prior live births, and typically happening before the 20th week of gestation. Both high and low concentrations of leptin have been attributed to recurrent miscarriages. Studies have explored the relationship between leptin levels and recurrent miscarriage, but the findings have been inconsistent. Some research has indicated that women with recurrent miscarriages may have higher leptin levels compared to those with normal pregnancies. Elevated leptin levels have been associated with conditions such as polycystic ovary syndrome (PCOS), which itself is linked to an increased risk of miscarriage. On the other hand, other studies have not found a significant difference in leptin levels between women with recurrent miscarriages and those with normal pregnancies. Additionally, there is limited evidence regarding the potential mechanisms through which leptin may influence miscarriage risk (Pérez-Pérez et al., 2018).

Gestational Diabetes Mellitus

Gestational diabetes mellitus (GDM) is characterized by spontaneous hyperglycemia during pregnancy and is the commonest metabolic complication that occurs in pregnant women with a high risk of maternal and perinatal morbidity (Soheilykhah et al., 2011; American Diabetes Association,

2018). International Diabetes Federation (IDF) in 2017 has approximated that 14% of pregnancies worldwide, representing approximately 18 million births annually, are being affected by GDM and its prevalence is higher in obese women (Powe et al., 2016). GDM is also associated with higher amounts of leptin and elevated expression of leptin receptors in the placenta. Apart from serum, higher leptin levels have also been measured in the amniotic fluid of women with GDM, with each 1 ng/dl rise in amniotic fluid leptin increasing the risk of developing GDM by 4% (Thagaard et al., 2017). The hyperinsulinemia seen in GDM stimulates leptin synthesis. Hence, the enhanced insulin resistance seen in GDM during the second half of pregnancy is also linked to higher leptin levels (De Gennaro et al., 2019). Macrosomic fetus (overweighed fetus) from diabetic mothers had higher umbilical cord leptin levels correlating with the fetal fat mass. Leptin may also contribute to the increased placental size seen in GDM (Pérez-Pérez et al., 2020). It is well established that leptin also plays a role in the functioning of immune system and leptin stimulates the release of inflammatory cytokines and increased placental leptin has been corresponded with a higher production of inflammatory cytokines IL-6 and TNF-α and correlated with the chronic inflammatory state observed in GDM. IL-6 and TNF-α also in turn regulate the placental expression of leptin (Gainsford et al., 1996; Al-Badri et al., 2015; De Gennaro et al., 2019).

Endometriosis

Endometriosis is an inflammatory disorder in which the endometrium, the tissue lining the uterus, develops outside the uterus, usually in the pelvic region (Kalaitzopoulos et al., 2020). With the incidence of 5 to 10%, it primarily affects females of reproductive age (Zondervan et al., 2018). Leptin has been linked to the emergence and spread of endometriosis. Endometriotic cells have been found to over-secrete leptin, which may speed up the development of endometriosis by increasing the release of inflammatory and angiogenic cytokines along with matrix metalloproteinases (Nácul et al., 2013). Leptin levels have been found to be higher in endometriosis-affected women, which may help to promote the growth and survival of endometrial tissue outside the uterus. A meta-analysis carried out by Kalaitzopoulos and coworkers (2021), demonstrated elevated leptin levels in the peritoneal fluid and follicular fluid of endometriosis-affected women in comparison to controls; these differences were not seen in the serum or plasma. The data discussed above disapprove of leptin's use as a blood diagnostic marker while suggesting a potential pathophysiologic significance for it in the neighborhood microenvironment.

Dysfunctional Labor

Dysfunctional or prolonged labor occurs when the duration of labor, particularly in the first stage, is extended beyond the normal range. Diagnosing delayed labor requires thorough monitoring of various factors, including the intensity, duration, and frequency of uterine contractions, as well as the progress of cervical dilation and descent of the fetus through the pelvis. The role of leptin in dysfunctional labor is not certain. Women who experienced a failed induction of labor (IOL) exhibited elevated levels of leptin in their maternal plasma. Additionally, these women had a higher likelihood of being obese and requiring multiple induction methods. The increased leptin values in conjunction with obesity may contribute to the failure of IOL in these cases (Cowman et al., 2022). The exact mechanisms by which leptin influences labor are not fully understood. It is believed that leptin may interact with other hormones and signaling pathways involved in uterine contraction and cervical ripening. Dysregulation of leptin signaling may disrupt the coordination and strength of uterine contractions, leading to dysfunctional labor. However, no significant correlation was found between leptin levels and the duration of the active phase of labor in non-obese women (Carlhäll et al., 2018).

Preterm Labor

Although leptin concentrations have been associated with prolonged labor in certain cases, mid-pregnancy (24-28 week) leptin level has been related with shortened gestation period (Branham et al., 2022). Higher leptin levels have been observed in women undergoing preterm labor (Huras et al., 2016). An experiment conducted on rats fed a high-fat diet demonstrated an elevation in leptin-induced uterine contractility, indicating an enhanced vulnerability to preterm labor (Pavithra et al., 2022). Other reports, however, indicate correlation of lower serum levels of leptin with preterm labor (Fakor et al., 2016). One proposed mechanism is that leptin may stimulate the release of inflammatory mediators, such as cytokines and prostaglandins, which are involved in the initiation of labor.

Leptin in Male Reproduction

The actions of leptin on male reproductive system have been studied less compared to female reproductive system. However, recent works from different authors suggest that leptin can act at different levels of the hypothalamic-pituitary-testicular axis. The major functions of leptin in male reproduction are still unclear due to the controversial and contradictory results shown by several research works. Most of them, if not all, indicate the negative effects of leptin on male reproduction. Leptin receptors are expressed in the Leydig and testicular germ cells in rats and mice (Zamorano et al., 1997; El-Hefnawy et al., 2000; Caprio et al., 2003) and in seminiferous tubules in humans (Glander et al., 2002; Ishikawa et al., 2007). Leptin receptors are also reported from interstitium and seminiferous tubules in pigs and leptin is implicated to participate in sperm capacitation through its receptors in acrosome of pig spermatozoa (De Ambrogi et al., 2007). Similar to females, leptin is required for attainment of puberty in males also as suggested by a dose dependant increase in pulsatile GnRH secretion following leptin administration in prepubertal male rats (Parent et al., 2000). Treatment of mice lacking leptin gene (Ob/Ob mice) with leptin resulted in elevated serum FSH levels, testicular and seminal vesicle weights and sperm count (Barash et al., 1996). Elevated levels of leptin as seen in obesity attenuated the gonadotropin-mediated testosterone secretion in cultured rat Leydig cells and a Leydig tumor cell lines (Caprio et al., 1999; Caprio et al., 2001; Tena-Sempere et al., 1999). Higher serum leptin levels are correlated with low androgen levels, low sperm count, testicular oxidative stress, high rate of morphological abnormalities and DNA fragmentation in sperm in obese men (Caprio et al., 2001; Haron et al., 2010; Almabhouh et al., 2015; Sengupta et al., 2019). This explains the direct correlation between reduced testosterone levels in hyperleptinaemic obese men. Subnormal amounts of testosterone in obese men may result in delayed onset and maintenance of sperm production, leading to fertility problems (Landry et al., 2013). Rats administered with exogenous leptin at 5 to 30 µg/kg body weight had lower seminiferous tubular epithelial height and diameter than similar aged healthy rats (Haron et al., 2010). Oxidative stress produced as a result of generation of ROS may increase sperm damage in seminiferous tubules or in the epididymis (Malik et al., 2019). Leptin can also pass through the mouse blood-testes barrier, enter the seminiferous tubules, and can impair mouse sperm development and the components of the blood-testis barrier (Banks et al., 1999, Wang et al., 2018). Childs and coworkers reported that there was lower sperm counts (by 50.9%)

and motility along with abnormal morphology in mice treated with 3 mg/kg leptin for 2 weeks and there was leakiness in the blood-testes barrier by reducing tight junction proteins (occludin, claudin 5 and Zonula Occudins-1) (Childs et al., 2021). Martins and co-workers studied the effect of leptin on isolated human Sertoli cells in culture which are very much essential for the physical and nutritional support of spermatogenesis by forming acetate from glucose. And they reported that physiological concentration of leptin increased glucose transporter 2 (GLUT2) proteins indicating normal leptin levels may help in spermatogenesis, whereas, obese levels of leptin produced a dose-dependent decrease in acetate production, indicating impaired Sertoli cell function in obese men (Martins et al., 2015).

Conclusion

In conclusion, leptin plays a significant role in reproductive health and may have implications in various reproductive diseases. Its involvement in regulating energy balance and body weight is closely tied to reproductive processes such as fertility, puberty onset, and pregnancy. Leptin levels and its receptors have been found in reproductive tissues, and dysregulation of leptin signaling has been associated with conditions such as polycystic ovary syndrome (PCOS), infertility, and preterm labor. While our understanding of leptin's exact mechanisms in reproductive health and diseases is still evolving, continued research holds promise for improving our knowledge and developing potential therapeutic interventions in the future. Further investigation into leptin's complex interactions within the reproductive system will shed light on its clinical significance and potential applications in managing reproductive disorders.

Funding

Nil

Declaration of interest

The authors declare that they have no known competing financial interests or personal relationships that could have appeared to influence the work reported in this chapter.

References

Achache, Hanna, Ariel Revel. Endometrial receptivity markers, the journey to successful embryo implantation. *Human Reproduction Update* (2006) 12(6):731-746.
Ahima R S, Dushay J, Flier S N, Prabakaran D, Flier J S. Leptin accelerates the onset of puberty in normal female mice. *The Journal of Clinical Investigation* (1997) 99(3):391-395.
Ahima R S, Flier J S. Leptin. *Annual Review of Physiology* (2000) 62(1):413-437.
Al-Badri MR, Zantout MS, Azar ST. The role of adipokines in gestational diabetes mellitus. *Therapeutic Advances in Endocrinology & Metabolism* (2015) 6(3):103-108.
Almabhouh F A, Osman K, Siti Fatimah I, Sergey G, Gnanou J, Singh H J. Effects of leptin on sperm count and morphology in Sprague-Dawley rats and their reversibility following a 6-week recovery period. *Andrologia* (2015) 47(7):751-758.
American Diabetes Association. 2. Classification and diagnosis of diabetes: standards of medical care in diabetes - 2018. *Diabetes Care* (2018) 41(Supplement_1):S13-S27.
Anderson C M, Lopez F, Zhang H Y, Pavlish K, Benoit J N. Characterization of changes in leptin and leptin receptors in a rat model of preeclampsia. *American Journal of Obstetrics & Gynecology* (2005) 193(1):267-272.
Anim-Nyame N, Sooranna S R, Steer P J, Johnson M R. Longitudinal analysis of maternal plasma leptin concentrations during normal pregnancy and pre-eclampsia. *Human Reproduction* (2000) 15(9):2033-2036.
Ashworth C J, Hoggard N, Thomas L, Mercer J G, Wallace J M, Lea R G. Placental leptin. *Reviews of Reproduction* (2000) 5(1):18-24.
Azziz R, Woods K S, Reyna R, Key T J, Knochenhauer ES, Yildiz BO. The prevalence and features of the polycystic ovary syndrome in an unselected population. *The Journal of Clinical Endocrinology & Metabolism* (2004) 89(6):2745-2749.
Bado A, Levasseur S, Attoub S, Kermorgant S, Laigneau J P, Bortoluzzi M N, Moizo L, Lehy T, Guerre-Millo M, Le Marchand-Brustel Y, Lewin M J. The stomach is a source of leptin. *Nature* (1998) 394(6695):790-793.
Baig M, Azhar A, Rehman R, Syed H, Tariq S, Gazzaz Z J. Relationship of serum leptin and reproductive hormones in unexplained infertile and fertile females. *Cureus* (2019) 1(12):e6524. doi: 10.7759/cureus.6524; PMID: 32025443; PMCID: PMC6991145.
Balogh O, Staub L P, Gram A, Boos A, Kowalewski M P, Reichler I M. Leptin in the canine uterus and placenta: possible implications in pregnancy. *Reproductive Biology & Endocrinology* (2015) 13(1):1-12.

Banks W A, McLay R N, Kastin A J, Sarmiento U, Scully S. Passage of leptin across the blood-testis barrier. *American Journal of Physiology-Endocrinology & Metabolism* (1999) 276(6):E1099-1104. doi: 10.1152/ajpendo.1999.276.6.E1099; PMID: 10362623.

Barash I A, Cheung C C, Weigle D S, Ren H, Kabigting E B, Kuijper J L, Clifton D K, Steiner R A. Leptin is a metabolic signal to the reproductive system. *Endocrinology* (1996) 137(7):3144-3147.

Barb C R. The brain-pituitary-adipocyte axis: role of leptin in modulating neuroendocrine function. *Journal of Animal Science* (1999) 77(5):1249-57.

Bates S H, Myers M G. The role of leptin receptor signaling in feeding and neuroendocrine function. *Trends in Endocrinology & Metabolism* (2003) 14(10):447-452.

Bates S H, Myers M G. The role of leptin→ STAT3 signaling in neuroendocrine function: an integrative perspective. *Journal of Molecular Medicine* (2004) 82:12-20.

Baumann H, Morella K K, White D W, Dembski M, Bailon P S, Kim H, Lai C F, Tartaglia L A. The full-length leptin receptor has signaling capabilities of interleukin 6-type cytokine receptors. *Proceedings of the National Academy of Sciences* (1996) 93(16):8374-8278.

Behboudi-Gandevani S, Ramezani Tehrani F, Bidhendi Yarandi R, Noroozzadeh M, Hedayati M, Azizi F. The association between polycystic ovary syndrome, obesity, and the serum concentration of adipokines. *Journal of Endocrinological Investigation* (2017) 40:859-866.

Bischof P, Meisser A, Campana A. Mechanisms of endometrial control of trophoblast invasion. *Journal of Reproduction & Fertility Supplement* (2000) 55:65-71.

Blum W F. Leptin: the voice of the adipose tissue. *Hormone Research in Paediatrics* (1997) 48(Suppl. 4):2-8.

Bogacka I, Przala J, Siawrys G, Kaminski T, Smolinska N. The expression of short form of leptin receptor gene during early pregnancy in the pig examined by quantitative real time RT-PCR. *Journal of Physiology & Pharmacology* (2006) 57(3):479-489.

Branham K A, Sherman E, Golzy M, Drobnis E Z, Schulz L C. Association of serum leptin at 24–28 weeks gestation with initiation and progression of labor in women. *Scientific Reports* (2022) 12(1):16016. doi: 10.1038/s41598-022-19868-0; PMID: 36163455; PMCID: PMC9512924.

Brannian J D, Hansen K A. "Leptin and ovarian folliculogenesis: implications for ovulation induction and ART outcomes". In *Seminars in Reproductive Medicine* (2002) 20(02):103-112. Copyright© 2002 by Thieme Medical Publishers, Inc., 333 Seventh Avenue, New York, NY 10001, USA. Tel.:+ 1 (212) 584-4662.

Brzechffa P R, Jakimiuk A J, Agarwal S K, Weitsman S R, Buyalos R P, Magoffin D A. Serum immunoreactive leptin concentrations in women with polycystic ovary syndrome. *The Journal of Clinical Endocrinology & Metabolism* (1996) 81(11):4166-4169. doi: 10.1210/jcem.81.11.8923878; PMID: 8923878.

Briana D D, Malamitsi-Puchner A. Reviews: adipocytokines in normal and complicated pregnancies. *Reproductive Sciences* (2009) 16(10):921-937.

Broughton D E, Moley K H. Obesity and female infertility: potential mediators of obesity's impact. *Fertility & Sterility* (2017) 107(4):840-847.

Cai C, Shi F D, Matarese G, La Cava A. Leptin as clinical target. Recent Patents on *Inflammation & Allergy Drug Discovery* (2009) 3(3):160-166.
Cameo P, Bischof P, Calvo J C. Effect of leptin on progesterone, human chorionic gonadotropin, and interleukin-6 secretion by human term trophoblast cells in culture. *Biology of Reproduction* (2003) 68(2):472-477.
Cao R. Brakenhielm E, Wahlestedt C, Thyberg J, Cao Y. Leptin induces vascular permeability and synergistically stimulates angiogenesis with FGF-2 and VEGF. *Proceedings of the National Academy of Sciences* (2001) 98:6390-6395.
Caprio M, Isidori A M, Carta A R, Moretti C, Dufau ML, Fabbri A. Expression of functional leptin receptors in rodent Leydig cells. *Endocrinology* (1999) 140(11):4939-4947.
Caprio M, Fabbrini E, Isidori A M, Aversa A, Fabbri A. Leptin in reproduction. *Trends in Endocrinology & Metabolism* (2001) 12(2):65-72.
Caprio M, Fabbrini E, Ricci G, Basciani S, Gnessi L, Arizzi M, Carta A R, De Martino M U, Isidori A M, Frajese G V, Fabbri A. Ontogenesis of leptin receptor in rat Leydig cells. *Biology of Reproduction* (2003) 68(4):1199-1207.
Carlhäll S, Källén K, Thorsell A, Blomberg M. Maternal plasma leptin levels in relation to the duration of the active phase of labor. *Acta Obstetricia et Gynecologica Scandinavica* (2018) 97(10):1248-1256.
Castellucci M, De Matteis R, Meisser A, Cancello R, Monsurro V, Islami D, Sarzani R, Marzioni D, Cinti S, Bischof P. Leptin modulates extracellular matrix molecules and metalloproteinases: possible implications for trophoblast invasion. *MHR: Basic Science of Reproductive Medicine* (2000) 6(10):951-958.
Cervero A, Horcajadas J A, Dominguez F, Pellicer A, Simon C. Leptin system in embryo development and implantation: a protein in search of a function. *Reproductive Biomedicine Online* (2005) 10(2):217-223.
Challier J, Galtier M, Bintein T, Cortez A, Lepercq J, Hauguel-de Mouzon S. Placental leptin receptor isoforms in normal and pathological pregnancies. *Placenta* (2003) 24(1):92-99.
Chehab F F, Mounzih K, Lu R, Lim M E. Early onset of reproductive function in normal female mice treated with leptin. *Science* (1997) 275(5296):88-90.
Cheung C C, Thornton J E, Kuijper J L, Weigle D S, Clifton D K, Steiner R A. Leptin is a metabolic gate for the onset of puberty in the female rat. *Endocrinology* (1997) 138(2):855-858. doi: 10.1210/endocr/bqaa204; PMID: 33165520; PMCID: PMC7749705.
Chen X, Jia X, Qiao J, Guan Y, Kang J. Adipokines in reproductive function: a link between obesity and polycystic ovary syndrome. *Journal of Molecular Endocrinology* (2013) 50(2):R21-37.
Childs G V, Odle A K, MacNicol M C, MacNicol A M. The importance of leptin to reproduction. *Endocrinology* (2021) 162(2):bqaa204. doi: 10.1210/endocr/bqaa204; PMID: 33165520; PMCID: PMC7749705.
Cioffi J A, Van Blerkom J, Antczak M, Shafer A, Wittmer S, Snodgrass H R. The expression of leptin and its receptors in pre-ovulatory human follicles. *Molecular Human Reproduction* (1997) 3(6):467-472.

Coleman D L. Obese and diabetes: two mutant genes causing diabetes-obesity syndromes in mice. *Diabetologia* (1978) 14:141-148.

Corvinus F M, Fitzgerald J S, Friedrich K, Markert U R. Evidence for a correlation between trophoblast invasiveness and STAT3 activity. *American Journal of Reproductive Immunology* (2003) 50(4):316-321.

Cowman W, Scroggins S M, Hamilton W S, Karras A E, Bowdler N C, Devor E J, Santillan M K, Santillan D A. Association between plasma leptin and cesarean section after induction of labor: a case control study. *BMC Pregnancy & Childbirth* (2022) 22(1):29. doi: 10.1186/s12884-021-04372-6; PMID: 35031012; PMCID: PMC8759283.

Coya R, Martul P, Algorta J, Aniel-Quiroga M A, Busturia M A, Señarís R. Effect of leptin on the regulation of placental hormone secretion in cultured human placental cells. *Gynecological Endocrinology* (2006) 22(11):620-626.

Craig J A, Zhu H, Dyce P W, Wen L, Li J. Leptin enhances porcine preimplantation embryo development in vitro. *Molecular & Cellular Endocrinology* (2005) 229(1-2):141-147.

De Ambrogi M, Spinaci M, Galeati G, Tamanini C. Leptin receptor in boar spermatozoa. *International Journal of Andrology* (2007) 30(5):458-461.

De Gennaro G, Palla G, Battini L, Simoncini T, Del Prato S, Bertolotto A, Bianchi C. The role of adipokines in the pathogenesis of gestational diabetes mellitus. *Gynecological Endocrinology* (2019) 35(9):737-751.

de Knegt V E, Hedley P L, Kanters J K, Thagaard I N, Krebs L, Christiansen M, Lausten-Thomsen U. The role of leptin in fetal growth during pre-eclampsia. *International Journal of Molecular Sciences* (2021) 22(9):4569. doi: 10.3390/ijms22094569; PMID: 33925454; PMCID: PMC8123779.

Demerath E W, Towne B, Wisemandle W, Blangero J, Cameron Chumlea W, Siervogel M. Serum leptin concentration, body composition, and gonadal hormones during puberty. *International Journal of Obesity* (1999) 23(7):678-685.

Dos Santos E, Serazin V, Morvan C, Torre A, Wainer R, de Mazancourt P, Dieudonné M N. Adiponectin and leptin systems in human endometrium during window of implantation. *Fertility & Sterility* (2012) 97(3):771-778.

Dyer C J, Simmons J M, Matteri R L, Keisler D H. Leptin receptor mRNA is expressed in ewe anterior pituitary and adipose tissues and is differentially expressed in hypothalamic regions of well-fed and feed-restricted ewes. *Domestic Animal Endocrinology* (1997) 14(2):119-128.

Ebihara K, Ogawa Y, Isse N, Mori K, Tamura N, Masuzaki H, Kohno K I, Yura S, Hosoda K, Sagawa N, Nakao K. Identification of the human leptin 5′-flanking sequences involved in the trophoblast-specific transcription. *Biochemical & Biophysical Research Communications* (1997) 241(3):658-663.

El-Hefnawy T, Ioffe S, Dym M. Expression of the leptin receptor during germ cell development in the mouse testis. *Endocrinology* (2000) 141(7):2624-2630.

Escobar-Morreale H F, San Millán J L. Abdominal adiposity and the polycystic ovary syndrome. *Trends in Endocrinology & Metabolism* (2007) 18(7):266-272.

Frühbeck G, Jebb S A, Prentice A M. Leptin: physiology and pathophysiology. *Clinical Physiology* (1998) 18(5):399-419.

Frühbeck G. Intracellular signalling pathways activated by leptin. *Biochemical Journal* (2006) 393(1):7-20.
Fakor F, Sharami S H, Milani F, Mirblouk F, Kazemi S, Pourmarzi D, Ebrahimi H, Heirati S F. The association between level of maternal serum leptin in the third trimester and the occurrence of moderate preterm labor. *Journal of the Turkish German Gynecological Association* (2016) 17(4):182. doi: 10.5152/jtgga.2016.16121; PMID: 27990085; PMCID: PMC5147755.
Fontana V A, Sanchez M, Cebral E, Calvo J C. Interleukin-1β regulates metalloproteinase activity and leptin secretion in a cytotrophoblast model. *Biocell* (2010) 34(1):37-43.
Gainsford T, Willson T A, Metcalf D, Handman E, McFarlane C, Ng A, Nicola N A, Alexander W S, Hilton D J. Leptin can induce proliferation, differentiation, and functional activation of hemopoietic cells. *Proceedings of the National Academy of Sciences* (1996) 93(25):14564-14568.
Garcia M R, Amstalden M, Williams S W, Stanko R L, Morrison C D, Keisler D H, Nizielski S E, Williams G L. Serum leptin and its adipose gene expression during pubertal development, the estrous cycle, and different seasons in cattle. *Journal of Animal Science* (2002) 80(8):2158-2167.
Glander H J, Lammert A, Paasch U, Glasow A, Kratzsch J. Leptin exists in tubuli seminiferi and in seminal plasma. *Andrologia* (2002) 34(4):227-233.
González R R, Caballero-Campo P, Jasper M, Mercader A, Devoto L, Pellicer A, Simon C. Leptin and leptin receptor are expressed in the human endometrium and endometrial leptin secretion is regulated by the human blastocyst. *The Journal of Clinical Endocrinology & Metabolism* (2000) 85(12):4883-4888.
Gonzalez R R, Leavis P C. A peptide derived from the human leptin molecule is a potent inhibitor of the leptin receptor function in rabbit endometrial cells. *Endocrine* (2003) 21:185-195.
Goumenou A G, Matalliotakis I M, Koumantakis G E, Panidis D K. The role of leptin in fertility. *European Journal of Obstetrics & Gynecology and Reproductive Biology* (2003) 106(2):118-124.
Gurugubelli Krishna R, Vishnu Bhat B. Molecular mechanisms of intrauterine growth restriction. *The Journal of Maternal-Fetal & Neonatal Medicine* (2018) 31(19):2634-2640.
Håkansson-Ovesjö M L, Collin M, Meister B. Down-regulated STAT3 messenger ribonucleic acid and STAT3 protein in the hypothalamic arcuate nucleus of the obese leptin-deficient (ob/ob) mouse. *Endocrinology* (2000) 141(11):3946-3955.
Haron M N, D'Souza U J, Jaafar H, Zakaria R, Singh H J. Exogenous leptin administration decreases sperm count and increases the fraction of abnormal sperm in adult rats. *Fertility & Sterility* (2010) 93(1):322-324.
Harrod J S, Rada C C, Pierce S L, England S K, Lamping K G. Altered contribution of RhoA/Rho kinase signaling in contractile activity of myometrium in leptin receptor-deficient mice. *American Journal of Physiology-Endocrinology & Metabolism* (2011) 301(2):E362-E369. PMID: 21558549; PMCID: PMC3154528.
Hoggard N, Hunter L, Duncan J S, Williams L M, Trayhurn P, Mercer J G. Leptin and leptin receptor mRNA and protein expression in the murine fetus and placenta. *Proceedings of the National Academy of Sciences* (1997) 94(20):11073-11078.

Hummel K P, Dickie M M, Coleman D L. Diabetes, a new mutation in the mouse. *Science* (1966) 153:1127-1128.

Huras H, Spaczyńska J, Gadamer A, Radoń-Pokracka M. An influence of changes in the levels of leptin on the risk of preterm delivery in patients with excessive BMI. *Przeglad Lekarski* (2016) 73(5):293-295.

Hynes G R, Jones P J. Leptin and its role in lipid metabolism. *Current Opinion in Lipidology* (2001) 12(3):321-327.

Ishikawa T, Fujioka H, Ishimura T, Takenaka A, Fujisawa M. Expression of leptin and leptin receptor in the testis of fertile and infertile patients. *Andrologia* (2007) 39(1):22-27.

Jaiswar S P, Priyadarshini A. Leptin and female reproductive health. (2021)

Kalaitzopoulos D R, Lempesis I G, Athanasaki F, Schizas D, Samartzis E P, Kolibianakis E M, Goulis D G. Association between vitamin D and endometriosis: a systematic review. *Hormones* (2020) 19:109-121.

Kalaitzopoulos D R, Lempesis I G, Samartzis N, Kolovos G, Dedes I, Daniilidis A, Nirgianakis K, Leeners B, Goulis D G, Samartzis E P. Leptin concentrations in endometriosis: A systematic review and meta-analysis. *Journal of Reproductive Immunology* (2021) 146:103338. doi: 10.1016/j.jri.2021.103338; PMID: 34126469.

Kalra S P. Mandatory neuropeptide-steroid signaling for the preovulatory luteinizing hormone-releasing hormone discharge. *Endocrine Reviews* (1993) 14(5):507-538.

Karlsson C, Lindell K, Svensson E, Bergh C, Lind P, Billig H, Carlsson L M, Carlsson B. Expression of functional leptin receptors in the human ovary. *The Journal of Clinical Endocrinology & Metabolism* (1997) 82(12):4144-4148.

Kawamura K, Sato N, Fukuda J, Kodama H, Kumagai J, Tanikawa H, Shimizu Y, Tanaka T. Survivin acts as an antiapoptotic factor during the development of mouse preimplantation embryos. *Developmental Biology* (2003) 256(2):331-341.

Kaynard A H, PAU K Y, Hess D L, Spies H G. Third-ventricular infusion of neuropeptide Y suppresses luteinizing hormone secretion in ovariectomized rhesus macaques. *Endocrinology* (1990) 127(5):2437-2444.

Kelesidis T, Kelesidis I, Chou S, Mantzoros C S. Narrative review: the role of leptin in human physiology: emerging clinical applications. *Annals of Internal Medicine* (2010) 152(2):93-100.

Kimber W, Peelman F, Prieur X, Wangensteen T, O'Rahilly S, Tavernier J, Farooqi I S. Functional characterization of naturally occurring pathogenic mutations in the human leptin receptor. *Endocrinology* (2008) 149(12):6043-6052.

Kitawaki J, Koshiba H, Ishihara H, Kusuki I, Tsukamoto K, Honjo H. Expression of leptin receptor in human endometrium and fluctuation during the menstrual cycle. *The Journal of Clinical Endocrinology & Metabolism* (2000) 85(5):1946-1950.

Kline A D, Becker G W, Churgay L M, Landen B E, Martin D K, Muth WL, Rathnachalam R, Richardson J M, Schoner B, Ulmer M, Hale J E. Leptin is a four-helix bundle: secondary structure by NMR. *FEBS letters* (1997) 407(2):239-242.

Kwon O, Kim K W, Kim M S. Leptin signalling pathways in hypothalamic neurons. *Cellular & Molecular Life Sciences* (2016) 73:1457-1477.

Löffler S, Aust G, Köhler U, Spanel-Borowski K. Evidence of leptin expression in normal and polycystic human ovaries. *Molecular Human Reproduction* (2001) 7(12):1143-1149. doi: 10.1093/molehr/7.12.1143; PMID: 11719591.

Landry D, Cloutier F, Martin L J. Implications of leptin in neuroendocrine regulation of male reproduction. *Reproductive Biology* (2013) 13(1):1-4.

Lappas M, Yee K, Permezel M, Rice G E. Release and regulation of leptin, resistin and adiponectin from human placenta, fetal membranes, and maternal adipose tissue and skeletal muscle from normal and gestational diabetes mellitus-complicated pregnancies. *Journal of Endocrinology* (2005) 186(3):457-465.

Lin J, Barb C R, Matteri R L, Kraeling R R, Chen X, Meinersmann R J, Rampacek G B. Long form leptin receptor mRNA expression in the brain, pituitary, and other tissues in the pig. *Domestic Animal Endocrinology* (2000) 19(1):53-61.

Lin J, Richard Barb C, Kraeling R R, Rampacek G B. Developmental changes in the long form leptin receptor and related neuropeptide gene expression in the pig brain. *Biology of Reproduction* (2001) 64(6):1614-1618.

Liu L L, Qiao J, Wang Y Z, Chen Y J, Gao Y Q. Expression of leptin and leptin receptor system in woman reproductive organs. *Zhonghua yi xue za zhi* (2003) 83(8):666-668.

Münzberg H, Björnholm M, Bates S H, Myers M G. Leptin receptor action and mechanisms of leptin resistance. *Cellular & Molecular Life Sciences* (2005) 62:642-652.

Münzberg H, Morrison C D. Structure, production and signaling of leptin. *Metabolism* (2015) 64(1):13-23.

Maamra M, Bidlingmaier M, Postel-Vinay M C, Wu Z, Strasburger C J, Ross R J. Generation of human soluble leptin receptor by proteolytic cleavage of membrane-anchored receptors. *Endocrinology* (2001) 142(10):4389-4393.

Madej T, Boguski M S, Bryant S H. Threading analysis suggests that the obese gene product may be a helical cytokine. *FEBS letters* (1995) 373(1):13-18.

Malik I A, Durairajanayagam D, Singh H J. Leptin and its actions on reproduction in males. *Asian Journal of Andrology* (2019) 21(3):296-299. doi: 10.4103/aja.aja_98_18; PMID: 30539926; PMCID: PMC6498734.

Martín-Romero C, Sánchez-Margalet V. Human leptin activates PI3K and MAPK pathways in human peripheral blood mononuclear cells: possible role of Sam68. *Cellular Immunology* (2001) 212(2):83-91.

Martins A D, Moreira A C, Sá R, Monteiro M P, Sousa M, Carvalho R A, Silva B M, Oliveira P F, Alves M G. Leptin modulates human Sertoli cells acetate production and glycolytic profile: a novel mechanism of obesity-induced male infertility?. *Biochimica et Biophysica Acta (BBA)-Molecular Basis of Disease* (2015) 1852(9):1824-1832.

Masuzaki H, Ogawa Y, Sagawa N, Hosoda K, Matsumoto T, Mise H, Nishimura H, Yoshimasa Y, Tanaka I, Mori T, Nakao K. Nonadipose tissue production of leptin: leptin as a novel placenta-derived hormone in humans. *Nature Medicine* (1997) 3(9):1029-1033. doi: 10.1038/nm0997-1029. PMID: 9288733.

Morash B, Li A, Murphy P R, Wilkinson M, Ur E. Leptin gene expression in the brain and pituitary gland. *Endocrinology* (1999) 140(12):5995-5998.

Morrison C D, Daniel J A, Hampton J H, Buff P R, McShane T M, Thomas M G, Keisler D H. Luteinizing hormone and growth hormone secretion in ewes infused intracerebroventricularly with neuropeptide Y. *Domestic Animal Endocrinology* (2003) 24(1):69-80.

Moynihan A T, Hehir M P, Glavey S V, Smith T J, Morrison J J. Inhibitory effect of leptin on human uterine contractility in vitro. *American Journal of Obstetrics & Gynecology* (2006) 195(2):504-509.

Mumtaz S, AlSaif S, Wray S, Noble K. Inhibitory effect of visfatin and leptin on human and rat myometrial contractility. *Life Sciences* (2015) 125:57-62.

Murakami T, Yamashita T, Iida M, Kuwajima M, Shima K. A short form of leptin receptor performs signal transduction. *Biochemical & Biophysical Research Communications* (1997) 231(1):26-29.

Nácul A P, Lecke S B, Edelweiss M I, Morsch D M, Spritzer P M. Gene expression of leptin and long leptin receptor isoform in endometriosis: a case-control study. *Obstetrics & Gynecology International* (2013) 2013:879618. doi: 10.1155/2013/879618; PMID: 23634146; PMCID: PMC3619696.

Nakamura S, Nishii N, Yamanaka A, Kitagawa H, Asano M, Tsubota T, Suzuki M. Leptin receptor (ob-R) expression in the ovary and uterus of the wild Japanese black bear (*Ursus thibetanus japonicus*). *Journal of Reproduction & Development* (2009) 55(2):110-115.

Nanjappa V, Raju R, Muthusamy B, Sharma J, Thomas J K, Nidhina P A, Harsha H C, Pandey A, Anilkumar G, Prasad T K. A comprehensive curated reaction map of leptin signaling pathway. *Journal of Proteomics & Bioinformatics* (2011) 4(9):181-189.

Nieuwenhuis D, Pujol-Gualdo N, Arnoldussen IA, Kiliaan A J. Adipokines: a gear shift in puberty. *Obesity Reviews* (2020) 21(6):e13005. doi: https://doi.org/10.1111/obr.13005; PMID: 32003144; PMCID: PMC7317558.

Ozata M, Ozdemir I C, Licinio J. Human leptin deficiency caused by a missense mutation: multiple endocrine defects, decreased sympathetic tone, and immune system dysfunction indicate new targets for leptin action, greater central than peripheral resistance to the effects of leptin, and spontaneous correction of leptin-mediated defects. *The Journal of Clinical Endocrinology & Metabolism*. (1999) 84(10):3686-3695.

Pérez-Pérez A, Maymó J, Dueñas J L, Goberna R, Calvo J C, Varone C, Sánchez-Margalet V. Leptin prevents apoptosis of trophoblastic cells by activation of MAPK pathway. *Archives of Biochemistry & Biophysics* (2008) 477(2):390-395.

Pérez-Pérez A, Maymó J, Gambino Y, Dueñas J L, Goberna R, Varone C, Sánchez-Margalet V. Leptin stimulates protein synthesis-activating translation machinery in human trophoblastic cells. *Biology of Reproduction* (2009) 81(5):826-832.

Pérez-Pérez A, Gambino Y, Maymó J, Goberna R, Fabiani F, Varone C, Sánchez-Margalet V. MAPK and PI3K activities are required for leptin stimulation of protein synthesis in human trophoblastic cells. *Biochemical & Biophysical Research Communications* (2010) 396(4):956-960.

Pérez-Pérez A, Sánchez-Jiménez F, Maymó J, Dueñas J L, Varone C, Sánchez-Margalet V. Role of leptin in female reproduction. *Clinical Chemistry & Laboratory Medicine (CCLM)* (2015) 53(1):15-28.

Pérez-Pérez A, Toro A, Vilariño-García T, Maymó J, Guadix P, Duenas J L, Fernández-Sánchez M, Varone C, Sánchez-Margalet V. Leptin action in normal and pathological pregnancies. *Journal of Cellular & Molecular Medicine* (2018) 22(2):716-727.

Pérez-Pérez A, Vilariño-García T, Guadix P, Dueñas J L, Sánchez-Margalet V. Leptin and nutrition in gestational diabetes. *Nutrients* (2020) 12(7):1970. doi: 10.3390/nu12071970; PMID: 32630697; PMCID: PMC7400219.

Parent A S, Lebrethon M C, Gerard A, Vandersmissen E, Bourguignon J P. Leptin effects on pulsatile gonadotropin releasing hormone secretion from the adult rat hypothalamus and interaction with cocaine and amphetamine regulated transcript peptide and neuropeptide Y. *Regulatory Peptides* (2000) 92(1-3):17-24.

Pavithra S, Kumar D K, Ramesh G, Panigrahi M, Sahoo M, Singh T U, Madhu C L, Manickam K, Shyamkumar T S, Kumar D, Parida S. Fat augments leptin-induced uterine contractions by decreasing JAK2 and BKCa channel expressions in late pregnant rats. *Cytokine* (2022) 157:155966. doi: 10.1016/j.cyto.2022.155966; PMID: 35905625.

Pennington K A, Oestreich A K, Cataldo K H, Fogliatti C M, Lightner C, Lydon J P, Schulz LC. Conditional knockout of leptin receptor in the female reproductive tract reduces fertility due to parturition defects in mice. *Biology of Reproduction* (2022) 107(2):546-556.

Plowden T C, Zarek S M, Rafique S, Sjaarda L A, Schisterman EF, Silver R M, Yeung E H, Radin R, Hinkle S N, Galai N, Mumford S L. Preconception leptin levels and pregnancy outcomes: A prospective cohort study. *Obesity Science & Practice* (2020) 6(2):181-188.

Pollheimer J, Knöfler M. Signalling pathways regulating the invasive differentiation of human trophoblasts: a review. *Placenta* (2005) 26:S21-30.

Powe C E, Allard C, Battista M C, Doyon M, Bouchard L, Ecker J L, Perron P, Florez J C, Thadhani R, Hivert M F. Heterogeneous contribution of insulin sensitivity and secretion defects to gestational diabetes mellitus. *Diabetes Care* (2016) 39(6):1052-1055.

Prolo P, Wong ML, Licinio J. Leptin. *The International Journal of Biochemistry & Cell Biology* (1998) 30(12):1285-1290. doi: 10.1016/s1357-2725(98)00094-6. PMID: 9924798.

Qian H, Barb C R, Compton M M, Hausman GJ, Azain MJ, Kraeling RR, Baile CA. Leptin mRNA expression and serum leptin concentrations as influenced by age, weight, and estradiol in pigs. *Domestic Animal Endocrinology* (1999) 16(2):135-143.

Quennell JH, Howell CS, Roa J, Augustine RA, Grattan DR, Anderson GM. Leptin deficiency and diet-induced obesity reduce hypothalamic kisspeptin expression in mice. *Endocrinology* (2011) 152(4):1541-1550.

Rosenblum C I, Tota M, Cully D, Smith T, Collum R, Qureshi S, Hess J F, Phillips M S, Hey P J, Vongs A, Fong TM. Functional STAT 1 and 3 signaling by the leptin receptor (OB-R); reduced expression of the rat fatty leptin receptor in transfected cells. *Endocrinology* (1996) 137(11):5178-5181.

Señarís R, Garcia-Caballero T, Casabiell X, Gallego R, Castro R, Considine RV, Dieguez C, Casanueva FF. Synthesis of leptin in human placenta. *Endocrinology* (1997) 138(10):4501-4504.

Sanchez-Jimenez F, Perez-Perez A, Gonzalez-Yanes C, Varone C L, Sanchez-Margalet V. Sam68 mediates leptin-stimulated growth by modulating leptin receptor signaling in human trophoblastic JEG-3 cells. *Human Reproduction* (2011) 26(9):2306-2315.

Sánchez-Jiménez F, Pérez-Pérez A, González-Yanes C, Najib S, Varone C L, Sánchez-Margalet V. Leptin receptor activation increases Sam68 tyrosine phosphorylation and expression in human trophoblastic cells. *Molecular & Cellular Endocrinology* (2011) 332(1-2):221-227.

Sanchez-Margalet V, Martin-Romero C. Human leptin signaling in human peripheral blood mononuclear cells: activation of the JAK-STAT pathway. *Cellular Immunology* (2001) 211(1):30-36.

Sengupta P, Bhattacharya K, Dutta S. Leptin and male reproduction. *Asian Pacific Journal of Reproduction* (2019) 8(5):220-226.

Serazin V, Duval F, Wainer R, Ravel C, Vialard F, Molina-Gomes D, Dieudonne M N, Dos Santos E. Are leptin and adiponectin involved in recurrent pregnancy loss?. *Journal of Obstetrics & Gynaecology Research* (2018) 44(6):1015-1022.

Sharif E, Rizk N M. Leptin And Free Leptin Receptor Is Associated With Polycystic Ovary Syndrome In Young Women. *International Journal of Endocrinology* (2015) 2015:927805. doi: 10.1155/2015/927805; PMID: 26180527; PMCID: PMC4477211.

Shimizu H, Shimomura Y, Nakanishi Y, Futawatari A, Ohtani K, Sato N, Mori M. Estrogen increases in vivo leptin production in rats and human subjects. *Journal of Endocrinology* (1997) 154(2):285-292.

Smolinska N, Siawrys G, Kaminski T, Przala J. Leptin gene and protein expression in the trophoblast and uterine tissues during early pregnancy and the oestrous cycle of pigs. *Journal of Physiology & Pharmacology* (2007) 58(3):563-581 PMID: 17928651.

Soheilykhah S, Mojibian M, Rahimi-Saghand S, Rashidi M, Hadinedoushan H. Maternal serum leptin concentration in gestational diabetes. *Taiwanese Journal of Obstetrics & Gynecology* (2011) 50(2):149-153.

Sosa C, Carriquiry M, Chalar C, Crespi D, Sanguinetti C, Cavestany D, Meikle A. Endometrial expression of leptin receptor and members of the growth hormone-Insulin-like growth factor system throughout the estrous cycle in heifers. *Animal Reproduction Science* (2010) 122(3-4):208-214.

Srinivasan G, Parida S, Pavithra S, Panigrahi M, Sahoo M, Singh T U, Madhu C L, Manickam K, Shyamkumar T S, Kumar D, Mishra S K. Leptin receptor stimulation in late pregnant mouse uterine tissue inhibits spontaneous contractions by increasing NO and cGMP. *Cytokine* (2021) 137:155341. doi: 10.1016/j.cyto.2020.155341; PMID: 33128919.

Sullivan S D, Moenter S M. γ-Aminobutyric acid neurons integrate and rapidly transmit permissive and inhibitory metabolic cues to gonadotropin-releasing hormone neurons. *Endocrinology* (2004) 145(3):1194-1202.

Tartaglia L A. The leptin receptor. *Journal of Biological Chemistry* (1997) 272(10):6093-6096.

Tena-Sempere M, Pinilla L, Gonzalez L C, Dieguez C, Casanueva F F, Aguilar E. Leptin inhibits testosterone secretion from adult rat testis in vitro. *Journal of Endocrinology* (1999) 161:211-218.

Thagaard I N, Krebs L, Holm J C, Lange T, Larsen T, Christiansen M. Adiponectin and leptin as first trimester markers for gestational diabetes mellitus: a cohort study. *Clinical Chemistry & Laboratory Medicine (CCLM)* (2017) 55(11):1805-1812.

Thomas M G, Gazal O S, Williams G L, Stanko R L, Keisler D H. Injection of neuropeptide Y into the third cerebroventricle differentially influences pituitary secretion of luteinizing hormone and growth hormone in ovariectomized cows. *Domestic Animal Endocrinology* (1999) 16(3):159-169.

Vázquez M J, Romero-Ruiz A, Tena-Sempere M. Roles of leptin in reproduction, pregnancy and polycystic ovary syndrome: consensus knowledge and recent developments. *Metabolism* (2015) 64(1):79-91.

Wang X, Zhang X, Hu L, Li H. Exogenous leptin affects sperm parameters and impairs blood testis barrier integrity in adult male mice. *Reproductive Biology & Endocrinology* (2018) 16:1-11.

Wauters M, Considine R V, Van Gaal L F. Human leptin: from an adipocyte hormone to an endocrine mediator. *European Journal of Endocrinology* (2000) 143(3):293-311.

Zamorano P L, Mahesh V B, De Sevilla L M, Chorich L P, Bhat G K, Brann D W. Expression and localization of the leptin receptor in endocrine and neuroendocrine tissues of the rat. *Neuroendocrinology* (1997) 65(3):223-228.

Zhang, Y. Proencar, Maffei M, Barone M, Leopold L, Friedman J M. Positional cloning of the mouse obese gene and its human homologue. *Nature* 372 (1994):425-432.

Zhang F, Basinski M B, Beals J M, Briggs S L, Churgay L M, Clawson D K, DiMarchi R D, Furman T C, Hale J E, Hsiung H M, Schoner B E. Crystal structure of the obese protein Ieptin-E100. *Nature* (1997) 387(6629):206-209.

Zidan H E, Rezk N A, Alnemr A A, Moniem M I. Interleukin-17 and leptin genes polymorphisms and their levels in relation to recurrent pregnancy loss in Egyptian females. *Immunogenetics* (2015) 67:665-673.

Zondervan K T, Becker C M, Koga K, Missmer S A, Taylor R N, Viganò P. Endometriosis (Primer). *Nature Reviews: Disease Primers* (2018) 4(1):9. doi: 10.1038/s41572-018-0008-5; PMID: 30026507.

Chapter 5

The Role of Leptin in Diabetes and Its Complications

Xiaoyu Xu[1]
Yigang Feng[2]
Cheng Zhang[1]
Ning Wang[1]
and Yibin Feng[1,*]

[1]School of Chinese Medicine, Li Ka Shing Faculty of Medicine, the University of Hong Kong, Hong Kong, China
[2]Guanghua School of Stomatology, Hospital of Stomatology, Sun Yat-sen University, Guangzhou, China

Abstract

Leptin is an important adipokine that is implicated in regulating energy metabolism and appetite to control food intake. However, the serum level of leptin is influenced by various factors, such as diet, lifestyle, and health conditions. The excess of leptin could lead to oxidative stress, inflammation, and angiogenesis, which can stimulate the development of diabetes and its complications. Moreover, elevated leptin levels are often observed in individuals with insulin resistance in both type 1 and type 2 diabetes, which can cause the body to become less responsive to insulin-regulating effects, leading to the accumulation of blood glucose. Furthermore, an imbalance in leptin levels can also stimulate endothelial dysfunction, angiogenesis, and oxidative stress, which are linked to the progression of several diabetic complications, including cardiovascular

---

* Corresponding Author's Email: yfeng@hku.hk.

In: Leptin and its Role in Health and Disease
Editor: Stephen E. Bradley
ISBN: 979-8-89113-274-0
© 2024 Nova Science Publishers, Inc.

disease, nephropathy, and retinopathy. In this chapter, we discuss the role of leptin in the pathogenesis and progression of diabetes and diabetic complications and the potential treatment via the regulation of leptin.

Keywords: diabetes, insulin resistance, diabetic complications

Introduction

Diabetes mellitus has a high prevalence all over the world and shows the tendency to occur at an earlier age, increasing the risk of premature death. Diabetes is generally classified into three types, namely, type 1 diabetes mellitus (T1DM), type 2 diabetes mellitus (T2DM), as well as gestational diabetes mellitus (GDM). The are differentiated by the charactistics of insulin deficiency, insulin resistance, and high blood sugar during pregnancy, respectively [1]. Diabetes mellitus is considered as a serious health concern due to the short- and long-term diabetic complications that patients suffer, such as diabetic retinopathy, foot ulcer, nephropathy, neuropathy, and cardiovascular diseases. As the prevalence and incidence of diabetes and its complications continue to rise, it is crucial to gain a better understanding of diseases' pathogenesis and potential treatment. This understanding will help in the development of new therapies and investigations in improving patient outcomes [2].

Leptin, an important hormone derived from adipose tissue, is implicated in the modulation of glucose metabolism and maintenance of energy balance. As the hormone primarily derived from the adipocytes in white adipose tissue, leptin could effectively control the food intake by modulating the appetite [3]. Increasing evidence proved that leptin has influence on the insulin sensitivity and the abnormal leptin level that can lead to endocrine disorders and increase the risk of obesity and diabetes. In addition, the leptin level is not only associated with the appetite regulation but involved in the stimulation of oxidative stress, inflammation, thrombosis, arterial stiffness, angiogenesis and atherogenesis, which promotes the pathogenesis of diabetic complications [4]. Given the impact of leptin on glucose metabolism and the development of diabetes, there is growing interest in the possibility of using leptin therapeutically to treat patients with diabetes.

In this chapter, we illuminate the role of leptin in the prevention and treatment of diabetes and its complications and its possible treatment like natural bioactive compounds according to the literature of the last five years.

This updated review may expand our knowledge of the health benefits and functions of leptin, as well as the promising approach to treating diabetes and its complications by regulating leptin levels.

Leptin and Type I Diabetes Mellitus

Since adipokines are strongly linked with insulin sensitivity and inflammation, the altered leptin level is considered as a main contributor to the pathogenesis of T1DM [5]. A case-control study including 133 type 1 diabetic children and 71 healthy controls displayed that leptin was significantly increased in the children with type 1 diabetes and was strongly correlated with HbA1c and BMI ($r = 0.245$, $p = 0.005$ and $r = 0.393$, $p < 0.001$ respectively), which indicated that the leptin may influence the insulin sensitivity [6]. Additionally, a prospective observational cohort study with 66 women with T1DM found a strong correlation between BMI and maternal blood leptin concentration. The gain of body mass was a main factor for the increased level of leptin in maternal blood, and meanwhile, the fat body mass was mainly related to the leptin levels in the neonate [7]. However, there is still some inconsistency about the change in serum leptin levels in patients with T1DM. A study reported that the increased leptin level showed no significant relationship in normal and diabetic children, while the correlation between resistin levels and the pathophysiology of T1DM, mediated through inflammation, was evident from the significant association between resistin levels and Hb1Ac levels [5].

In the animal models of T1DM at an earlier stage, the endogenous leptin levels are relatively low. Thus, leptin treatment could exert glucose-lowering effects on STZ-induced T1DM mice fed with standard diet [7]. In addition, the cross-mated insulin-deficient mice with leptin-expressing transgenic mice displayed the normal glycemic control and maintained insulin hypersensitivity as well as the glucose tolerance. The results demonstrated the therapeutic efficacy of leptin for long-term treatment of insulin-deficient diabetes in mice [8] However, under the more humanized physiological conditions like having high-fat diets, the adiposity and the leptin resistance were induced in mice, which largely eliminated the glucose-lowering effects of leptin [7]. Notably, most patients with T1DM also showed a high level of leptin level and they were often treated with insulin therapy meanwhile, and thus, the effects of leptin were indicated to be associated with other factors like plasma glucagon and gluconeogenesis rather than plasma insulin [7]. Moreover, it was stated that the treatment of leptin mediated the later parabrachial nucleus to respond to hypoglycemia in uncontrolled diabetes, which further inhibited the secretion of glucagon and the ketosis [9]. Although the leptin has the glucose-lowering effect, a very high level of exogenous leptin seems to be ineffective in eliciting a significant response in leptin-resistant animals or humans. The application of leptin in lowering glucose level in patients with T1DM may be limited.

Leptin and Type II Diabetes Mellitus

T2DM is characterized by the insulin resistance and needs a very high dose of insulin to control the blood glucose. Leptin is hypothesized as the product of obesity-related genes and works as a main attributor to the regulation of body weight, indicating its potential in treating obesity and T2DM. A clinical study including 71 patients with T2DM and 32 controls found that the mRNA level of leptin was remarkedly reduced in diabetic patients, and the level of leptin exhibited a significant correlation with blood glucose and glycosylated haemoglobin, with AUC values of 0.88 and 0.97, respectively, indicating that the mRNA expression level of leptin serves as the predictive biomarker for T2DM development [10]. In a cross-sectional study detected in 39 patients with T2DM, the results demonstrated that the patients with T2DM had lower levels of leptin and the leptin receptor gene polymorphism, which influenced the glucose metabolism by modulating the insulin resistance and the function of pancreatic beta cells and further affect the pathogenesis of T2DM [11]. In the zebrafish model, the deficiency of *lepb*, the gene encoding leptin, caused a high level of blood glucose and the obesity and as well as the early signs of diabetic nephropathy. It indicated that leptin deficiency affected glucose homeostasis and could lead to the adiposity in zebrafish [12]. These findings suggested that obese animals or people had a relatively low level of endogenous leptin, and the leptin therapy might be effective in losing body weight, but the likelihood of a response to leptin diminished at an increasingly higher leptin level [13].

On the other hand, elevated endogenous leptin levels are commonly observed in most forms of obesity and obesity-related complications like T2DM in both animals and patients, with reduced response to exogenous hormone and the development of leptin resistance as the disease progresses [14]. The affinity kinetics assays showed that the leptin-reactive immunoglobulins (IgG) displayed lower binding capacity and affinity to leptin in obese T2DM patients, indicating the leptin resistance [15]. In addition, an observational study resulted that the serum leptin level was significantly associated with the obesity index. The serum leptin level was increased in patients with T2DM and obesity. There were significant positive correlations between the level of leptin and that of fasting glucose, total cholesterol (TC), low-density Lipoprotein (LDL) cholesterol and very low-density lipoprotein (VLDL) cholesterol, while it was negatively correlated with the level of high-density lipoprotein (HDL) cholesterol [16]. These findings illustrated a controversy with the aforementioned results, suggesting that leptin therapy is of limited value in the treatment of T2DM. It is acknowledged that leptin functions in regulating the energy homeostasis by suppressing appetite and reducing the adipose tissue mass as well as the body weight. The lean animals have a lower leptin level and could reduce the body weight via leptin therapy. Hence, the leptin therapy may be effective at the earlier stage of T2DM when the leptin level is still low. However, the obese animals showed a higher endogenous level of leptin and became leptin resistant, which the leptin therapy malfunctions in T2DM treatment [17, 18].

Leptin is also strongly linked with the other impairment induced by T2DM. Serum leptin levels and leptin resistance are strongly related to the pathophysiology of NAFLD in patients with T2DM. The hepatic steatosis was found to have a positive correlation with serum leptin and leptin resistance, and negatively with the concentration of leptin receptor sObR, but neither of leptin related indexes made a significant contribution to hepatic fibrosis [19]. As leptin is a critical regulator of the reproductive system that targets hypothalamic-pituitary-gonadal axis, abnormal testicular leptin signalling may contribute to the impaired male reproductive function during the progression of T2DM. Male rats with T2DM exhibited reduced plasma testosterone levels, decreased sperm counts, and abnormal sperm morphology, likely due to severe metabolic progression, hormonal imbalances and dysregulated testicular leptin signaling [20]. Additionally, the cross-sectional studies resulted that the serum leptin levels were enhanced, and the ratio of resting energy expenditure to leptin was reduced in T2DM patients with depression and anxiety symptoms, which indicated that the development of depression and anxiety symptoms was related to the increased leptin levels and leptin resistance in patients with T2DM [21].

The function of leptin in T2DM is also mediated by other factors. Neurotensin in central nervous system is involved in the regulatory effects of leptin on appetite and energy homeostasis, and its circulating level is associated with the progression of obesity and T2DM. The leptin level was correlated with the high level of pro-neurotensin and thus, the neurotensin might modulate the energy metabolism via the leptin level and the potential mechanism was implicated with the gut fat absorption in T2DM [22]. Irisin is a novel exercise-regulated myokine that is proposed to induce "browning" or "beigeing" in white adipose tissue and regulate the energy homeostasis, which is regarded as the potential agent for treating diabetes and obesity [23]. Thus, the levels of irisin and leptin in obesity and insulin resistance have gained research focuses recently. A nested case-control study demonstrated that obese individuals display higher leptin concentrations regardless of their glucose tolerance, while obese individuals with impaired glucose tolerance had higher levels of irisin [23].

Leptin and Gestational Diabetes Mellitus

Leptin is expressed at high level by the trophoblastic cells in the placenta, which is responsible for the important autocrine trophic effects. The leptin levels were also increased in patients with GDM, the most frequent pathology of pregnancy [24]. In early pregnancy, the maternal circulating leptin and ratio of leptin/adiponectin ratio were significantly altered and increased the risk of developing GDM in pregnant women, suggesting that the hyperleptinemia might be a predictor for GDM [25, 26]. And the leptin levels went high at the early pregnancy but increased slightly in the late pregnancy, indicating that the compensatory response to intensifying insulin resistance was disturbed in GDM patients during the pregnancy [25]. Additionally, the high level of leptin in plasma might promote the leptin resistance at the central level, and the obesity-induced inflammation was also a main contributor to leptin resistance in GDM. Hence, the nutritional intervention is the primary approach for preventing and treating of GDM [27]. Leptin was also found to be positively correlated with the level of aquaporin 9 in GDM patients, suggesting that aquaporin 9 could be a predictor of the abnormal maternal metabolic environment for GDM [28]. Moreover, the progression of diabetes during pregnancy increased the level of IL-6 which could further promote the leptin production. The pathogenesis of maternal diabetes and birth weight were associated with leptin levels, and the neuroprotective effects of leptin were limited due to the increased cord blood level of IL-6 with potential neurotoxin in the term infant and placenta [29]. In addition to its effects on mothers, exposure to GDM can have impacts on offspring health. GDM induced a higher leptin level in GDM offspring than that in controls and potentially promote metabolic disorders as well as higher obesity prevalence among

GDM offspring [30]. However, some studies demonstrated that there was no significant difference in leptin level among obese and DM mothers as well as lean mothers. Thus, the change in leptin level may not represent the altered maternal metabolic environment in pregnant women with diabetes and obesity [31].

Leptin and Diabetic Complications

Neuropathy is a frequent diabetic complication with severe consequences as the disease progresses and largely affects the whole-body systems [32]. The elevated levels of HOMA-IR, leptin and resistin had been identified as the risk factors for diabetic nephropathy in T2DM patients with lower BMI rather than those with obesity [33]. The deficiency of leptin receptor could lead to abnormal pathological changes in intervertebral disc degeneration (IVDD) and cell apoptosis, and notably, these effects of leptin were sex-dependent in the spine, particularly for females [34, 35]. Proteomic quantitative study showed that proteins were expressed differentially in peripheral nerves in mice with T2DM compared to the controls, which the energetic deficiency was identified as the primary mechanism underlying neurodegeneration in diabetic neuropathy [36]. Moreover, the pathology of Alzheimer's Disease (AD) is partly due to the disruption of insulin signaling and homeostasis, and the leptin could greatly influence the function of hippocampus. The oral intake of a leptin mimetic synthetic peptide could increase the efficacy of insulin on the level of blood glucose and improve the cognitive function in rats with T1DM. The combination of insulin and the leptin mimetic molecules was suggested to prevent the progression of AD by alleviating the memory disruption [37]. Furthermore, the serum leptin level had association with the severity and risk of stroke, and it was reduced in the patients with poor outcomes and nonsurvivors and exhibited a negative association with ischemic stroke in patients with T2DM [38].

Diabetes increases the risk of developing cardiovascular diseases, which is one of the most common complications, and the diabetic state is regarded as the main risk factor for micro- and macro-cardiovascular disease progression [39, 40]. A prospective study investigated the correlation between cardiovascular risk factors and T1DM in 175 diabetic children and 150 controls. It resulted that the pathology of T1DM increased the risk of impairing the carotid and aortic artery structure and function, which might further affect the arterial wall stiffening and thickening [39]. The high level of serum leptin was significantly associated with peripheral arterial stiffness (PAS) in T2DM patients, indicating that leptin level could be a predictor of PAS and the aortic dysfunction [41]. On the other hand, the expressions of leptin receptor and leptin were not significantly different in atherosclerotic plaque between DM patients and controls, while the number of leptin receptors tended to be increased in DM atherosclerotic plaques [42]. Statins are considered as potential drugs for preventing atherosclerotic cardiovascular complications in T2DM patients. The rosuvastatin ameliorated atherosclerotic cardiovascular diseases in dyslipidemic T2DM patients with a reduction in leptin levels [43].

The gastric emptying rate is influenced by acute changes in blood glucose levels, with acute hyperglycemia activating the gastric inhibitory vagal motor, while acute hypoglycemia activates the gastric excitatory vagal motor circuit and accelerates gastric emptying. Research suggests that the stomach can modulate the rate of emptying by producing certain gastric "braking" hormones, including leptin, which can help prevent rapid gastric emptying and better manage postprandial hyperglycemia [44]. Diabetes is present in about 45% to 65% of patients with pancreatic ductal adenocarcinoma (PDAC), and conversely, the data supported that diabetes enhanced the risk of PDAC [45]. Leptin as the adipokine was implicated to be involved in the development of obesity-associated diseases like PDAC. However, a prospective study with 56 PDAC patients and 56 controls elucidated that the serum leptin levels were not significantly correlated with the presence of PDAC and survival, suggesting that leptin level might not be the regulator for the prognostic role of diabetes in PDAC [46].

Treatment of Diabetes and Its Complications via Leptin

Therapeutic attempts to control the glycaemia and treat diabetic complications have been a long-term issue for research. The aggerate data supports that nutritional intervention like a healthy lifestyle and intake of natural compounds could improve diabetes and its complication via the regulation of leptin. Physical training is a common but important factor that influences the energy homeostasis and leptin levels. Aerobic exercise training and resistance exercise training reduced the level of serum leptin in diabetic rats with T2DM, but the de-training could eliminate these benefits like increasing the leptin level after 4 weeks [47]. In addition, the aerobic training reduced leptin levels and improved the insulin resistance by regulating the function of leptin not irisin in young obese men with T2DM [48]. However, the aerobic training or short-term physical activity failed to alter the leptin levels in T2DM patients with diabetic neuropathy [49]. Thus, the effect of short-term physical training is limited on diabetes and its complications, while long-term physical training could improve the metabolic disorders by normalizing leptin levels.

Due to the low toxicity and limited side effects, natural compounds are receiving increasing attention as potential options for preventing and treating diabetes and its associated complication. Ginsenoside Rb1, the major bioactive components from *Panax ginseng* and *Panax notoginseng* ameliorated obesity, diabetes and its complications by regulating glycolipid metabolism and improving the insulin and leptin sensitivities due to its potent antioxidant, anti-inflammatory and anti-apoptosis effects [50]. A polyphenolic compounds from *Corni Fructus*, 7-O-galloyl-D-sedoheptulose, exerted anti-diabetic effects of mice with T2DM by reducing the leptin level, oxidative stress and inflammation [51]. Moreover, *Antrodia camphorate*, a rare parasitic fungus, could dose-dependently reduce the serum leptin and insulin levels and improve the insulin resistance in T2DM, which might be involved in the modulation of TNF-α, IL-6 and PPARγ [52].

Other nutritional supplement, natural hormone, and anti-diabetic drugs are used in the treatment by regulating the leptin levels. Patients with T2DM displayed a deficiency of coenzyme Q10 (CoQ10), and the supplementation of CoQ10 in women patients with T2DM could decrease the leptin level and improve the leptin resistance [53]. The development of T2DM is often accompanied with neuroinflammation and the disturbance in indoleamine 2,3-dioxygenase 1 (IDO1). The findings illustrated that the treatment of melatonin ameliorated the altered metabolic profile and inflammation in T2DM, in which the leptin level was reduced. Melatonin also alleviated the brain oxidative stress, decreased the IDO1 expression in hippocampus and improved the neuronal morphology in the hippocampus of rats with HFD-induced T2DM [54]. Additionally, the amino acid compound containing a 7-(diethylamino) coumarin-3-carboxamide side-chain could prevent the diabetes and ameliorate the anxiety-related behavior by stimulating the leptin receptor LepR/PKCς/glucose transporter 1 (GLUT1) [55]. Dipeptidyl peptidase-4 inhibitors (DPP-4i) are a group of antihyperglycemic medications used to manage T2DM via incretin peptides. Linagliptin, a DPP-4i, and metformin could both ameliorate the HFD-induced elevated leptin level and improve the diabetic osteoporosis by modulating bone morphogenetic protein-2 (BMP-2) and sclerostin [56]. Sodium-glucose cotransporter-2 (SGLT2) inhibitors have been approved as the agent in T2DM treatment and showed potent anti-inflammatory effects. Its treatment could effectively reduce the level of leptin in T2DM subjects, alleviating the inflammation and protecting cardiorenal system [57].

Although some antidiabetic drugs can affect the leptin levels in patients, the clinical studies are still few and the mechanism remains uncertain to draw a conclusion about their effects on leptin, and extensive additional clinical validation is needed to demonstrate the role and potential of leptin as the therapeutic target in treatment of diabetes and its complications.

Conclusion

Leptin plays a crucial role in regulating appetite to control body weight and maintaining energy homeostasis. Numerous studies have linked leptin to the progression of diabetes, including T1DM, T2DM, GDM, and several associated complications. In most forms of diabetes, the serum leptin levels are high, and the leptin resistance is developed which eliminates the glucose-lowering effects of leptin on diabetes. Hence, the potential for leptin to act as a useful therapy in treating diabetes is constrained. Some treatments like physical training and natural compounds could ameliorate diabetes and its complications by regulating the leptin levels. Although anti-diabetic drugs may affect leptin levels, sufficient clinical evidence is lacking, and additional research is necessary to determine whether leptin could be a potential target in the therapies of diabetes and its complications.

References

[1] Saeedi P., Petersohn I., Salpea P., Malanda B., Karuranga S., Unwin N., Stephen Colagiuri, Leonor Guariguata, Ayesha A. Motala, Katherine Ogurtsova, Jonathan E. Shaw, Dominic Bright, Rhys Williams. (2019). Global and regional diabetes prevalence estimates for 2019 and projections for 2030 and 2045: Results from the international diabetes federation diabetes atlas, 9th edition. *Diabetes Research and Clinical Practice*, 157.

[2] Meek T. H. and Morton G. J. (2016). The role of leptin in diabetes: Metabolic effects. *Diabetologia*, 59(5): 928-932.

[3] Martinez-Sanchez N. (2020). There and back again: Leptin actions in white adipose tissue. *International Journal of Molecular Sciences*, 21(17).

[4] Katsiki N., Mikhailidis D. P., and Banach M. (2018). Leptin, cardiovascular diseases and type 2 diabetes mellitus. *Acta Pharmacologica Sinica*, 39(7): 1176-1188.

[5] Saboktakin L. (2020). Leptin and resistin levels in iranian children with type 1 diabetes mellitus. *Crescent Journal of Medical and Biological Sciences,* 7(3): 368-372.

[6] Huneif M. A., Shalayel M. H. F., Hassan E. E., Elhussein A. B., Fadlelseed O. E., Hamid H. G. M., Amin A. A. Elbadawi, Sultan A. Almedhesh, Seham M. Alqahtani, Abdulwahab Alqahtani, Mohammed Jamaan Alzahrani, Dhafer Batti Alshehri. (2022). The association between leptin levels with glycemic control, body mass index, and progression of hba1c values in type 1 diabetic children in southwestern saudi arabia. *Medical Science,* 26(120).

[7] Zouhar P., Rakipovski G., Bokhari M. H., Busby O., Paulsson J. F., Conde-Frieboes K. W., Johannes J. Fels, Kirsten Raun, Birgitte Andersen, Barbara Cannon, Jan Nedergaard. (2020). Ucp1-independent glucose-lowering effect of leptin in type 1 diabetes: Only in conditions of hypoleptinemia. *American Journal of Physiology-Endocrinology and Metabolism,* 318(1): E72-E86.

[8] Naito M., Fujikura J., Ebihara K., Miyanaga F., Yokoi H., Kusakabe T., Yuji Yamamoto, Cheol Son, Masashi Mukoyama, Kiminori Hosoda, Kazuwa Nakao. (2011). Therapeutic impact of leptin on diabetes, diabetic complications, and longevity in insulin-deficient diabetic mice. *Diabetes,* 60(9): 2265-2273.

[9] Meek T. H., Matsen M. E., Faber C. L., Samstag C. L., Damian V., Nguyen H. T., Jarrad M. Scarlett, Jonathan N. Flak, Martin G. Myers Jr, Gregory J. Morton. (2018). In uncontrolled diabetes, hyperglucagonemia and ketosis result from deficient leptin action in the parabrachial nucleus. *Endocrinology,* 159(4): 1585-1594.

[10] Al-Harithy R. N. and Alomari A. S. (2021). Expression of leptin mrna as non-invasive biomarker in type 2 diabetes mellitus. *International Journal of Clinical Practice,* 75(12).

[11] Adiga U., Banawalikar N., Mayur S., Bansal R., Ameera N., and Rao S. (2021). Association of insulin resistance and leptin receptor gene polymorphism in type 2 diabetes mellitus. *Journal of the Chinese Medical Association,* 84(4): 383-388.

[12] He J. L., Ding Y., Nowik N., Jager C., Eeza M. N. H., Alia A., Hans J. Baelde, Herman P. Spaink. (2021). Leptin deficiency affects glucose homeostasis and results in adiposity in zebrafish. *Journal of Endocrinology,* 249(2): 125-134.

[13] Friedman J. M. (2019). Leptin and the endocrine control of energy balance. *Nature Metabolism,* 1(8): 754-764.

[14] Maffei M., Halaas J., Ravussin E., Pratley R. E., Lee G. H., Zhang Y., H. Fei, S. Kim, R. Lallone, S. Ranganathan, P. A. Kern & J. M. Friedman. (1995). Leptin levels in human and rodent - measurement of plasma leptin and ob rna in obese and weight-reduced subjects. *Nature Medicine,* 1(11): 1155-1161.

[15] Bouhajja H., Bougacha-Elleuch N., Lucas N., Legrand R., Marrakchi R., Kaveri S. V., Kamel Jamoussi, Hammadi Ayadi, Mohamed Abid, Mouna Mnif-Feki, Serguei O. Fetissov. (2018). Affinity kinetics of leptin-reactive immunoglobulins are associated with plasma leptin and markers of obesity and diabetes. *Nutrition & Diabetes,* 8.

[16] Gawali R., Bahulikar A., Phalgune D. S., and Tambolkar A. (2019). Association between serum leptin levels obesity in and type 2 diabetes mellitus. *Journal of Clinical and Diagnostic Research,* 13(10).

[17] Halaas J. L., Boozer C., BlairWest J., Fidahusein N., Denton D. A., and Friedman J. M. (1997). Physiological response to long-term peripheral and central leptin infusion in lean and obese mice. *Proceedings of the National Academy of Sciences of the United States of America,* 94(16): 8878-8883.

[18] Peng X. M., Huang J. J., Zou H. J., Peng B., Xia S. S., Dong K., Nan Sun, Jing Tao, Yan Yang. (2022). Roles of plasma leptin and resistin in novel subgroups of type 2 diabetes driven by cluster analysis. *Lipids in Health and Disease,* 21(1).

[19] Cernea S., Roiban A. L., Both E., and Hutanu A. (2018). Serum leptin and leptin resistance correlations with nafld in patients with type 2 diabetes. *Diabetes-Metabolism Research and Reviews,* 34(8).

[20] Derkach K. V., Bakhtyukov A. A., Roy V., Gryaznov A. Y., Bayunova L. V., and Shpakov A. O. (2020). The testicular leptin system in rats with different severity of type 2 diabetes mellitus. *Journal of Evolutionary Biochemistry and Physiology,* 56(1): 22-30.

[21] Cernea S., Both E., Hutanu A., Sular F. L., and Roiban A. L. (2019). Correlations of serum leptin and leptin resistance with depression and anxiety in patients with type 2 diabetes. *Psychiatry and Clinical Neurosciences,* 73(12): 745-753.

[22] Barchetta I., Ciccarelli G., Cimini F. A., Ceccarelli V., Orho-Melander M., Melander O., M. G. Cavallo. (2018). Association between systemic leptin and neurotensin concentration in adult individuals with and without type 2 diabetes mellitus. *Journal of Endocrinological Investigation,* 41(10): 1159-1163.

[23] Sahin-Efe A., Upadhyay J., Ko B. J., Dincer F., Park K. H., Migdal A., Pantel Vokonas, Christos Mantzoros. (2018). Irisin and leptin concentrations in relation to obesity, and developing type 2 diabetes: A cross sectional and a prospective case-control study nested in the normative aging study. *Metabolism-Clinical and Experimental,* 79: 24-32.

[24] Peltokorpi A., Irina L., Liisa V., and Risto K. (2022). Preconceptual leptin levels in gestational diabetes and hypertensive pregnancy. *Hypertension in Pregnancy,* 41(1): 70-77.

[25] Xiao W. Q., He J. R., Shen S. Y., Lu J. H., Kuang Y. S., Wei X. L., Xiu Qiu. (2020). Maternal circulating leptin profile during pregnancy and gestational diabetes mellitus. *Diabetes Research and Clinical Practice,* 161.

[26] Bawah A. T., Seini M. M., Abaka-Yawason A., Alidu H., and Nanga S. (2019). Leptin, resistin and visfatin as useful predictors of gestational diabetes mellitus. *Lipids in Health and Disease,* 18(1).

[27] Perez-Perez A., Vilarino-Garcia T., Guadix P., Duenas J. L., and Sanchez-Margalet V. (2020). Leptin and nutrition in gestational diabetes. *Nutrients,* 12(7).

[28] Sezer S., Kaya S., Behram M., and Dag I. (2022). Increased maternal serum aquaporin 9 levels in pregnancies complicated with gestational diabetes mellitus. *Journal of Maternal-Fetal & Neonatal Medicine,* 35(1): 18-23.

[29] Vasilakos L. K., Steinbrekera B., Santillan D. A., Santillan M. K., Brandt D. S., Dagle D., Robert D. Roghair. (2022). Umbilical cord blood leptin and il-6 in the presence of maternal diabetes or chorioamnionitis. *Frontiers in Endocrinology,* 13.

[30] Kampmann F. B., Thuesen A. C. B., Hjort L., Bjerregaard A. A., Chavarro J. E., Frystyk J., Mette Bjerre, Inge Tetens, Sjurdur F. Olsen, Allan A. Vaag, Peter Damm,

Louise G. Grunnet. (2019). Increased leptin, decreased adiponectin and fgf21 concentrations in adolescent offspring of women with gestational diabetes. *European Journal of Endocrinology*, 181(6): 691-700.

[31] Johnson A. W., Snegovskikh D., Parikh L., DeAguiar R. B., Han C. S., and Hwang J. J. (2020). Characterizing the effects of diabetes and obesity on insulin and leptin levels amongst pregnant women. *American Journal of Perinatology*, 37(11): 1094-1101.

[32] Bharadwaj P., Wijesekara N., Liyanapathirana M., Newsholme P., Ittner L., Fraser P., Giuseppe Verdile. (2017). The link between type 2 diabetes and neurodegeneration: Roles for amyloid-beta, amylin, and tau proteins. *Journal of Alzheimers Disease*, 59(2): 421-432.

[33] Huang J. J., Peng X. M., Dong K., Tao J., and Yang Y. (2021). The association between insulin resistance, leptin, and resistin and diabetic nephropathy in type 2 diabetes mellitus patients with different body mass indexes. *Diabetes Metabolic Syndrome and Obesity-Targets and Therapy*, 14: 2357-2365.

[34] Natelson D. M., Lai A., Krishnamoorthy D., Hoy R. C., Iatridis J. C., and Illien-Junger S. (2020). Leptin signaling and the intervertebral disc: Sex dependent effects of leptin receptor deficiency and western diet on the spine in a type 2 diabetes mouse model. *Plos One*, 15(5).

[35] Li X. H., Liu X. M., Wang Y. R., Cao F. M., Chen Z. X., Hu Z. Y., Bin Yu, Hang Feng, Zhaoyu Ba, Tao Liu, Haoxi Li, Bei Jiang, Yufeng Huang, Lijun Li & Desheng Wu. (2020). Intervertebral disc degeneration in mice with type ii diabetes induced by leptin receptor deficiency. *Bmc Musculoskeletal Disorders*, 21(1).

[36] Leal-Julia M., Vilches J. J., Onieva A., Verdes S., Sanchez A., Chillon M., Xavier Navarro, Assumpció Bosch. (2022). Proteomic quantitative study of dorsal root ganglia and sciatic nerve in type 2 diabetic mice. *Molecular Metabolism*, 55.

[37] Anderson B. M., Hirschstein Z., Novakovic Z. M., and Grasso P. (2020). Ma- d-leu-4 -ob3, a small molecule synthetic peptide leptin mimetic, mirrors the cognitive enhancing action of leptin in a mouse model of type 1 diabetes mellitus and alzheimer's disease-like cognitive impairment. *International Journal of Peptide Research and Therapeutics*, 26(3): 1243-1249.

[38] Zou Y., Hu L., Zou W. J., and Li H. L. (2020). Association of low leptin with poor 3-month prognosis in ischemic stroke patients with type 2 diabetes. *Clinical Interventions in Aging*, 15: 2353-2361.

[39] Zhang Y., Zhang H., and Li P. (2019). Cardiovascular risk factors in children with type 1 diabetes mellitus. *Journal of Pediatric Endocrinology & Metabolism*, 32(7): 699-705.

[40] Aaty T. A. A., Rezk M. M., Megallaa M. H., Yousseif M. E., and Kassab H. S. (2020). Serum leptin level and microvascular complications in type 2 diabetes. *Clinical Diabetology*, 9(4): 239-244.

[41] Lu C. W., Lee C. J., Hou J. S., Wu D. A., and Hsu B. G. (2018). Positive correlation of serum leptin levels and peripheral arterial stiffness in patients with type 2 diabetes. *Tzu Chi Medical Journal*, 30(1): 10-14.

[42] Dimitrova D. A., Mikhailov I. A., Tokarev K. Y., Michurova M. S., Gorbacheva A. M., Danilova N. V., P. G. Malkov, V. Y. Kalashnikov. (2021). Leptin and leptin

receptor evaluation in atherosclerotic plaques in patients with type 2 diabetes mellitus. *Terapevticheskii Arkhiv*, 93(10): 1186-1192.

[43] Werida R., Khairat I., and Khedr N. F. (2021). Effect of atorvastatin versus rosuvastatin on inflammatory biomarkers and lv function in type 2 diabetic patients with dyslipidemia. *Biomedicine & Pharmacotherapy, 135*.

[44] Goyal R. K., Cristofaro V., and Sullivan M. P. (2019). Rapid gastric emptying in diabetes mellitus: Pathophysiology and clinical importance. *Journal of Diabetes and Its Complications*, 33(11).

[45] Kuang T. T., Jin D. Y., Wang D. S., Xu X. F., Ni X. L., Wu W. C., Wen Hui Lou. (2009). Clinical epidemiological analysis of the relationship between pancreatic cancer and diabetes mellitus: Data from a single institution in china. *Journal of Digestive Diseases,* 10(1): 26-29.

[46] Man T., Seicean R., Lucaciu L., Leucuta D., Ilies M., Iuga C., L. Petrusel, A. Seicean. (2022). Leptin involvement in the survival of pancreatic adenocarcinoma patients with obesity and diabetes. *European Review for Medical and Pharmacological Sciences*, 26(4): 1341-1349.

[47] Ghozhdi H. D., Heidarianpour A., Keshvari M., and Tavassoli H. (2021). Exercise training and de-training effects on serum leptin and tnf-alpha in high fat induced diabetic rats. *Diabetology & Metabolic Syndrome*, 13(1).

[48] Rezaeeshirazi R. (2022). Aerobic versus resistance training: Leptin and metabolic parameters improvement in type 2 diabetes obese men. *Research Quarterly for Exercise and Sport*, 93(3): 537-547.

[49] Molnar A., Szentpeteri A., Lorincz H., Seres I., Harangi M., Balogh Z., Péter Kempler, György Paragh, Ferenc Sztanek. (2022). Change of fibroblast growth factor 21 level correlates with the severity of diabetic sensory polyneuropathy after six-week physical activity. *Reviews in Cardiovascular Medicine*, 23(5).

[50] Zhou P., Xie W. J., He S. B., Sun Y. F., Meng X. B., Sun G. B., Xiaobo Sun. (2019). Ginsenoside rb1 as an anti-diabetic agent and its underlying mechanism analysis. *Cells*, 8(3).

[51] Park C. H., Noh J. S., Jeon J. P., and Yokozawa T. (2023). A systematic review on anti-diabetic action of 7-o-galloyl-d- sedoheptulose, a polyphenol from corni fructus, in type 2 diabetic mice with hepatic and pancreatic damage. *Drug Discoveries and Therapeutics*.

[52] Kuang Y., Chai Y., Su H. F., Lo J. Y., Qiao X., and Ye M. (2022). A network pharmacology-based strategy to explore the pharmacological mechanisms of antrodia camphorata and antcin k for treating type ii diabetes mellitus. *Phytomedicine*, 96.

[53] Gholami M., Zarei P., Sedeh B. S., Rafiei F., and Khosrowbeygi A. (2018). Effects of coenzyme q10 supplementation on serum values of adiponectin, leptin, 8-isoprostane and malondialdehyde in women with type 2 diabetes. *Gynecological Endocrinology*, 34(12): 1059-1063.

[54] Maher A. M., Saleh S. R., Elguindy N. M., Hashem H. M., and Yacout G. A. (2020). Exogenous melatonin restrains neuroinflammation in high fat diet induced diabetic rats through attenuating indoleamine 2,3-dioxygenase 1 expression. *Life Sciences*, 247.

[55] Lee A., Sun Y., Lin T., Song N. J., Mason M. L., Leung J. H., Devan Kowdley, Jennifer Wall, Alessandro Brunetti, Julie Fitzgerald, Lisa A. Baer, Kristin I. Stanford, Joana Ortega-Anaya, Laisa Gomes-Dias, Bradley Needleman, Sabrena Noria, Zachary Weil, Joshua J. Blakeslee, Rafael Jiménez-Flores, Jon R. Parquette, Ouliana Ziouzenkova. (2020). Amino acid-based compound activates atypical pkc and leptin receptor pathways to improve glycemia and anxiety like behavior in diabetic mice. *Biomaterials*, 239.

[56] Nirwan N. and Vohora D. (2022). Linagliptin in combination with metformin ameliorates diabetic osteoporosis through modulating bmp-2 and sclerostin in the high-fat diet fed c57bl/6 mice. *Frontiers in Endocrinology*, 13.

[57] Wang D. M., Liu J. Y., Zhong L., Li S. H., Zhou L. Y., Zhang Q., Ming Li, Xinhua Xiao. (2022). The effect of sodium-glucose cotransporter 2 inhibitors on biomarkers of inflammation: A systematic review and meta-analysis of randomized controlled trials. *Frontiers in Pharmacology*, 13.

Chapter 6

The Role of Leptin in Nutrition and Cancer

Hasan Gencoglu[1], PhD
and Kazim Sahin[2], PhD

[1]Department of Biology, Faculty of Science, Firat University, Elazig, Turkey
[2]Department of Animal Nutrition and Nutritional Disorders,
Faculty of Veterinary Medicine, Firat University, Elazig, Turkey

Abstract

Leptin is a hormone primarily secreted by adipose tissue that plays a crucial role in regulating energy homeostasis and feeding behavior. Understanding the role of leptin in cancer may provide insights into potential therapeutic targets for cancer treatment. Leptin signaling has been shown to promote cancer cell proliferation, angiogenesis, and invasiveness in several types of cancer, including breast, prostate, and colorectal cancer. Additionally, leptin has been shown to contribute to the resistance of cancer cells to chemotherapy and radiation therapy. However, the precise mechanisms underlying these effects of leptin on cancer development and progression are not yet fully understood. In addition to its well-known role in obesity and metabolic disorders, recent research has uncovered a potential link between leptin and cancer. This review summarizes the current understanding of the role of leptin in nutrition and cancer, focusing on its impact on cancer cell proliferation, angiogenesis, and immune response. Preclinical studies have demonstrated that inhibition of leptin signaling can suppress tumor growth and sensitize cancer cells to chemotherapy and radiation therapy. Clinical studies investigating the efficacy of targeting leptin signaling in cancer treatment are currently underway, and early results have shown promising results. Leptin signaling has been shown to activate various signaling pathways, including JAK/STAT, PI3K/Akt, and MAPK/ERK, which promote cancer cell growth and survival. Moreover, leptin can

In: Leptin and its Role in Health and Disease
Editor: Stephen E. Bradley
ISBN: 979-8-89113-274-0
© 2024 Nova Science Publishers, Inc.

modulate the tumor microenvironment by promoting angiogenesis and inhibiting immune response, facilitating tumor progression. However, conflicting results exist regarding the association between leptin levels and human cancer risk. Thus, further research is needed to elucidate the complex interplay between leptin and cancer fully. In conclusion, the role of leptin in nutrition and cancer is an active area of research, and emerging evidence suggests that targeting leptin signaling may be a promising therapeutic strategy for cancer. Further studies are needed to elucidate the precise mechanisms underlying the effects of leptin on cancer development and progression and to determine the optimal therapeutic approach for targeting leptin signaling in cancer treatment.

Keywords: cancer, leptin, molecular pathways, nutrition

Introduction

Leptin, discovered in 1994, emerged as a pivotal peptide hormone involved in the intricate interplay between energy balance, metabolism, and body weight regulation. Extensive research has revealed that leptin acts as a signaling molecule in various tissues and profoundly affects multiple physiological systems. Leptin is mainly synthesized and secreted by adipocytes, which also plays a critical role in energy homeostasis, metabolism, and regulation of various physiological processes (Dornbush and Aeddula 2023). A broad understanding of the hormone leptin is essential to unravel its multifaceted physiological roles and to explore potential therapeutic targets for metabolic disorders.

Leptin Hormone and General Characteristics

Leptin is synthesized as a 16-kDa protein precursor in adipocytes and undergoes post-translational modifications, including cleavage of the signal peptide, glycosylation, and formation of a disulfide bond. The mature form of leptin consists of 167 amino acids with a tertiary structure resembling that of the cytokine family, particularly interleukin-6. It binds to the long form of the leptin receptor (LEPR) located predominantly in the hypothalamus (Stępień et al., 2023; Obradovic et al., 2021). It is encoded by the ob gene and primarily secreted by adipose tissue. The release of leptin from adipocytes is tightly regulated by various factors, including nutritional status, adiposity, and hormonal signals. Increased adipose tissue mass results in elevated leptin levels, while fasting or reduced fat stores lead to decreased secretion. Other hormonal mediators, such as insulin and glucocorticoids, also influence leptin synthesis and release. Leptin secretion exhibits a diurnal rhythm, with levels peaking during the night. Upon binding to LEPR in the hypothalamus, leptin triggers a signaling cascade involving the Janus kinase (JAK)/signal transducer and activator of the transcription (STAT) pathway. This signaling pathway regulates the expression of neuropeptides, such as pro-opiomelanocortin (POMC) and agouti-related peptide (AgRP), which are key modulators of appetite and energy expenditure. Leptin activation of ObR also leads to the activation of the PI3K (Phosphoinositide 3-kinase)/Akt (Protein Kinase B)/mTOR (mammalian Target of Rapamycin) pathway as well (Savova et al., 2023) (Figure 1). Additionally, leptin influences the release of other neurotransmitters and hormones, such as melanocortins and thyroid-stimulating hormones, contributing to its overall metabolic effects (Varela and Horvath 2012; Ladyman and Grattan 2013).

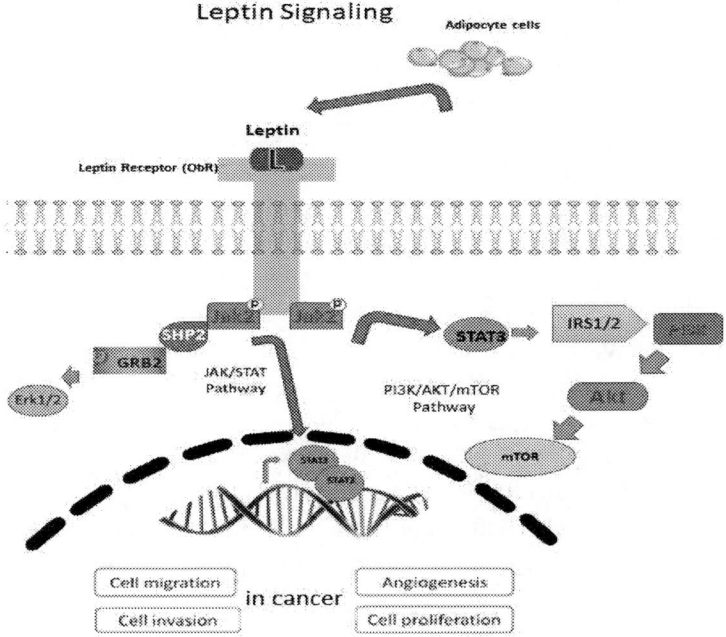

Figure 1. Leptin signaling in the mammalian cells. JAK2 (Janus kinase 2), SHP2 (Src homology 2 domain-containing protein tyrosine phosphatase 2), Grb2 (Growth factor receptor-bound protein 2), ERK1/2 (Extracellular signal-regulated kinase 1/2), STAT3 (Signal transducer and activator of transcription 3), IRS1 (Insulin receptor substrate 1), PI3K (Phosphatidylinositol 3-kinase), AKT (Protein kinase B), mTOR (Mammalian target of rapamycin).

Leptin plays a pivotal role in appetite regulation, serving as a satiety signal communicating the body's energy status to the brain. It acts as a negative feedback signal, reducing food intake and promoting energy expenditure. Additionally, leptin impacts reproductive function, as it influences gonadotropin-releasing hormone secretion and reproductive hormone levels (Park and Ahima 2015; Budak et al., 2006). Leptin also influences immune function by modulating inflammatory responses and regulating lymphocyte proliferation. Dysregulation of leptin signaling has been implicated in various pathological conditions, including obesity, insulin resistance, and reproductive disorders (Iikuni et al., 2008). Leptin exhibits a broad range of physiological effects encompassing appetite regulation, energy balance, reproduction, and immune function (Park and Ahima 2015). Through its complex signaling pathways, leptin plays a crucial role in maintaining energy homeostasis and metabolic equilibrium. Leptin has central effects that regulate energy balance and have an impact on a variety of processes in various tissues. Due to its primary function in maintaining homeostasis of energy, adipose tissue is a major target of leptin action via autocrine, paracrine, or endocrine signaling (Picó et al., 2022).

The brain, specifically the brainstem and hypothalamus, is where leptin primarily exerts its effects. The ventral tegmental region and the solitary tract are the brainstem's primary activity areas. Here, leptin influences satiety as well as the regulation of reward and aversion. The primary locations of leptin action in the hypothalamus are the ventromedial, dorsomedial, ventral pre-mammillary, and arcuate nuclei (ARC). The thyroid, gonadal, adrenocorticotropic hormone-cortisol growth hormone axes, as well as alterations in whole-brain cognition, emotion, memory, and structure, are all affected by the activation of these areas. Numerous of these connections are still being clarified. Further research is warranted to unravel the intricate mechanisms underlying leptin signaling and its potential therapeutic implications in managing metabolic disorders. A comprehensive understanding of leptin will continue to provide valuable insights into regulating energy balance and developing targeted interventions (Dornbush and Aeddula 2023).

Relationship of Leptin Hormone and Nutrition

Leptin acts as a vital feedback signal to the brain, alerting it about energy reserves and modifying energy intake and usage. Circulating levels of leptin are highly influenced by nutritional status, notably caloric intake and adipose tissue mass. higher adipose tissue results in higher leptin synthesis in energy-surplus conditions, such as obesity. On the other hand, leptin secretion is suppressed by energy restriction, such as fasting or reduced calorie consumption. Leptin levels and dietary status have a dynamic interaction that keeps energy homeostasis in check (Rosenbaum and Leibel 2014). The main way leptin regulates appetite is through altering the activity of hypothalamic neurons that control appetite. By inhibiting the release of orexigenic neuropeptides like neuropeptide Y (NPY) and Agouti-related protein (AgRP) and stimulating the release of anorexigenic neuropeptides like pro-opiomelanocortin (POMC)-derived peptides, increased leptin levels, reflecting sufficient energy stores, suppress appetite and promote satiety. On the other side, lower levels of leptin brought on by dietary restriction increase appetite and limit energy use, encouraging energy conservation.

Leptin therapy demonstrates its effectiveness in regulating glucose levels, body weight, and overall metabolic health when administered during a state of heightened leptin sensitivity. This sensitivity is commonly observed in leptin-deficient ob/ob mice, individuals with lipodystrophy, and a small subset of obese individuals. By reinstating leptin sensitivity within hypothalamic neurons, even in the presence of leptin resistance (often observed in diet-induced obesity, or as a consequence of genetic or pharmacological leptin reduction, either alone or in combination with other medications), significant benefits are observed, including reduced food intake, substantial weight loss, and improved insulin sensitivity. Additionally, interventions specifically targeting the reduction of leptin levels in the bloodstream have been shown to enhance insulin sensitivity (Zhao et al., 2020; Şener, Alver, and Cevher 2022).

The macronutrient composition of the diet can also influence leptin secretion and sensitivity. Studies have shown that high-fat diets increase leptin levels, possibly due to enhanced leptin synthesis by adipose tissue. Additionally, diets rich in carbohydrates, particularly those with a high glycemic index, have been associated with lower leptin levels and reduced leptin sensitivity. These findings suggest that the type and quality of macronutrients can modulate leptin signaling and contribute to changes in energy balance. Leptin interacts with various hormones involved in appetite regulation and energy metabolism. Insulin, for example, stimulates leptin secretion, and both hormones work together to regulate food intake and body weight. In conditions of insulin resistance, such as obesity and type 2 diabetes, impaired insulin signaling can disrupt the leptin-insulin axis, leading to leptin resistance and dysregulated appetite control. Additionally, ghrelin, a hormone secreted by the stomach, acts in opposition to leptin, stimulating hunger and food intake. The balance between leptin and ghrelin levels is crucial for maintaining energy balance and proper appetite regulation (Gencoglu et al., 2020; Gencoglu 2023; Orhan et al., 2022; Klok, Jakobsdottir, and Drent 2007).

Leptin Hormone and Cancer

Leptin has been the subject of research investigating its potential association with cancer development and progression. While the exact mechanisms are still being elucidated, several studies have examined the relationship between leptin and various types of cancers. Leptin, classified as a cytokine and considered a nutritional substance, plays a significant role in cancer progression. In obesity, the functions of leptin, which is secreted by adipocytes and acts as a hormone-like cytokine/adipokine, differ from its functions in a normal, healthy state. Elevated levels of leptin in obese individuals are associated with specific cancer types due to its pro-inflammatory adipokine properties. In recent years, several studies have been conducted to investigate changes in leptin levels among cancer patients, along with exploring the effects of various nutritional interventions (Table 1).

Epidemiological studies have revealed a direct association between obesity and cancer. Obesity increases the risk of cancer and related chronic diseases. Moreover, the imbalance of adipokines like leptin plays a significant role in neoplasm pathogenesis, cell migration, and consequently cancer metastasis. A recent meta-analysis identified the LEP gene rs7799039 and ADIPOQ gene rs1501299 as two potential candidate loci associated with an increased risk of breast cancer (Peng et al., 2023). Leptin has also been found to upregulate the levels of human epidermal growth factor receptor 2 (HER2) protein in breast cancer cells via the heat shock protein (Hsp90) STAT3-mediated pathway. Insulin and insulin-like growth factors (IGFs) have been identified as mitotic activators in both host and cancerous breast epithelial cells. Hyperinsulinemia explains the positive relationship between colorectal cancer and obesity. In prostate cancer, changes in sex hormone levels, such as testosterone and dihydrotestosterone, have been reported, along with increased oxidative stress, as the main contributors to tumor development. On the other hand, there are two interconnected factors that play a crucial role in the psychological loop related to lung cancer (Pandit et al., 2023).

Table 1. Some recent trial studies on leptin level changes in cancer patients

Study	Type	Main Methods	Main outcomes	Reference
Effects of decaffeinated green coffee extract (DGCE) supplementation on leptin	Randomized Controlled Trial	A total of 44 breast cancer patients aged between 18 and 70 years with obesity and a mean body mass index (BMI) of 31.62 ± 4.97 kg m -2 participated in this study. The treatment group (n = 22) and control group (n = 22) received two 400 mg decaffeinated green coffee extract (DGCE) capsules or two identical placebos daily for 12 weeks.	DGCE supplementation had no significant effect on leptin levels in breast cancer survivors with obesity.	(Bahmannia et al., 2022)
Effect of flaxseed on leptin in women with polycystic ovary syndrome	Randomized Controlled Trial	This randomized, open-labeled controlled clinical trial was conducted on 41 patients with Polycystic Ovary Syndrome. The participants were randomized to take either flaxseed powder (30 g/day) plus lifestyle modification or only lifestyle modification for 12 weeks.	Flaxseed supplementation led to a significant reduction in leptin compared with the control group.	(Haidari et al., 2020)
Antiestrogenic tamoxifen and toremifene levels in postmenopausal breast cancer patients	Clinical Trial	Thirty postmenopausal patients with breast cancer were randomized to start either with tamoxifen (20 mg/day, n=15) or toremifene (40 mg/day, n=15), and the patients were examined and serum leptin concentrations measured before the study and at 6 and 12 months.	Antiestrogens may stimulate the synthesis and release of leptin in the adipocytes.	(Marttunen et al., 2000)
Exercise-Induced Dose-Response Alterations in Adiponectin and Leptin	Randomized Controlled Trial	A 5-menstrual-cycle-long dosed aerobic exercise intervention compared low-dose exercise (150 min/wk; n = 44) or high-dose exercise (300 min/wk; n = 48) with a control group asked to maintain usual activity levels (n = 45). Exercise intensity progressed to and was maintained at 70% to 80% of age predicted heart rate max.	In this randomized clinical trial of premenopausal women at risk for breast cancer, we demonstrate a dose-response effect of exercise on adiponectin and leptin and that dose response is dependent on changes in body fat.	(Sturgeon et al., 2016)

Table 1. (Continued)

Study	Type	Main Methods	Main outcomes	Reference
Effect of coffee consumption on leptin levels in US health professionals	Clinical Trial	Data were derived from 2 cohorts of 15,551 women (Nurses' Health Study) and 7397 men (Health Professionals Follow-Up Study).	Compared with non-drinkers, participants who drank ≥4 cups of total coffee per day had lower leptin levels.	(Hang et al., 2019)
Leptin itself promotes the proliferation and migration of MDA-MB-231 breast cancer cells	Randomized Controlled Trial	MDA-MB-231 breast cancer cells were randomly divided into control group and (50, 100, 200, 400) ng/mL leptin treated groups. MDA-MB-231 cells and leptin receptor genes were silenced and the silenced cells were stimulated with different concentrations of leptin, then cell proliferation was detected by MTT assay, cell migration was detected by scratch assay was detected by Western blot.	Leptin up-regulates in MDA-MB-231 cells and promotes cell proliferation and migration.	(Zhou et al., 2022)
The effect of melatonin on leptin in the treatment of patients with non-alcoholic fatty liver disease	Randomized Controlled Trial	The study was conducted on 24 participants from the melatonin group and 21 participants from the placebo group. Participants took 1 mg of melatonin or placebo 6 hours before bedtime daily. The intervention period was 12 weeks.	6 mg/day melatonin administration had an improved effect on leptin serum levels.	(Bahrami et al., 2020)
Effect on Leptin PCOS Women of Levels in High Dosage Vitamin D	Randomized Controlled Trial	Ninety-nine women with polycystic ovary syndrome were randomized to 3 drug treatment arms: spironolactone (50 mg/d; n=30), metformin (1000 mg/d; n=) and pioglitazone (30 mg/d; n=30). These women also received oral vitamin D (4000 IU/d) and the allocated drug for 6 months.	Combining high-dose vitamin D with spironolactone or pioglitazone was more effective than metformin in reducing plasma leptin levels.	(Rashid et al., 2020)
Leptin levels in breast cancer survivors	Clinical Trial	A total of 136 breast cancer survivors with cancer-related fatigue were randomly allocated to the mindfulness acupuncture group and the control group in a 1:1 ratio, with 68 cases in each group.	Mental regulation acupuncture significantly reduced leptin levels in breast cancer survivors with cancer-related fatigue.	(Li et al., 2023)

Moreover, it has been suggested that poor prognostic factors may contribute to high concentrations of circulating leptin and increased expression of leptin receptors (Ob-R) in tumors. The exact mechanisms explaining how leptin is linked to unfavorable prognosis remain unclear, but there are various biological components associated with leptin that may contribute to tumor cell invasion and distant metastasis. These components include interactions with carcinoma-associated fibroblasts, the tumor-promoting effects of infiltrating macrophages, activation of matrix metalloproteinases, and signaling pathways such as transforming growth factor-β. Recent studies have also revealed leptin's involvement in epithelial-mesenchymal transition, a crucial phenomenon in cancer cell migration and metastasis. Additionally, there have been reports of leptin's synergistic effects with insulin-like growth factor-I, epidermal growth factor receptor, and HER2/neu. Leptin's impact on both adenocarcinomas and squamous cell carcinomas has been demonstrated in relation to an unfavorable prognosis (Ray and Cleary 2017).

It has been suggested that leptin, like insulin, acts as a growth factor for breast cancer cells. Breast cancer linked to obesity poses a serious risk, particularly to postmenopausal women. The microenvironment generated at the level of adipose tissue, which contains inflammatory cytokines, appears to be the basis of the association between obesity and breast cancer (Sánchez-Jiménez et al., 2019). Obesity has been positively associated with gastric cancer. The European Prospective Investigation into Cancer and Nutrition cohort reported in a very recent study that leptin levels were positively associated with non-cardiac gastric cancer in men (Sanikini et al., 2023). In patients with colorectal cancer, baseline values of leptin, visfatin, and resistin have been reported to serve as prognostic indicators for poor response to chemotherapy (Słomian et al., 2017). In a recent study on gallbladder cancer (GBC) was conducted in North India, involving 40 GBC patients and 40 healthy controls. It was found that serum leptin levels were significantly lower in GBC patients. No significant association was observed between serum leptin and cancer stage or tumor markers. A positive correlation was found between serum leptin and BMI in GBC patients. It is suggested that the lower serum leptin levels in GBC may be influenced by the patients' low BMI and appearance (Krishnan M P et al., 2023). In another recent study, researchers examined genetic variants of leptin and leptin receptor in CRC survival. They analyzed data from 532 CRC patients and found out that LEP and LEPR were associated with disease-free survival (DFS) and CRC-specific survival. While specific SNPs in LEP and LEPR were linked to DFS, certain LEPR haplotypes were associated with prolonged survival in CRC patients, particularly in colon cancer cases. Interactions were found between LEPR variants, red meat intake, BMI, and DFS. Polymorphic variations in LEP and LEPR genes were linked to CRC patient survival, influenced by red meat intake and BMI (Du et al., 2023).

Table 2. Key directions and applications for leptin and cancer therapy

Targeted Therapies	Developing targeted therapies that directly interfere with leptin signaling pathways to inhibit tumor growth and metastasis. This could involve the design of specific leptin receptor inhibitors or downstream signaling pathway blockers.
Combination Therapies	Exploring combination therapies that utilize leptin-targeting agents alongside existing cancer treatments to enhance their effectiveness and reduce treatment resistance.
Personalized Medicine	Investigating the potential of using leptin levels and leptin receptor expression as biomarkers for personalized cancer treatment. This could help identify patients who may benefit the most from leptin-targeted therapies.
Immunotherapy	Studying the interplay between leptin and the immune system in the context of cancer, and exploring the potential of immunotherapies that modulate leptin's effects on immune responses to improve cancer outcomes.
Nutritional Interventions	Evaluating the impact of nutritional interventions on leptin levels and its role in cancer prevention and treatment. This could include dietary modifications and supplements that influence leptin production and sensitivity.
Cancer Prevention	Investigating how leptin dysregulation contributes to cancer development and progression, with the aim of developing preventive strategies to mitigate cancer risk through leptin regulation.
Clinical Trials	Conducting well-designed clinical trials to assess the safety and efficacy of leptin-based therapies in various cancer types, providing essential data for potential approval and implementation in clinical practice.
Leptin Sensitizers	Identifying compounds or agents that enhance leptin sensitivity in cancer cells, potentially leading to new therapeutic approaches that exploit the body's natural regulatory mechanisms.
Leptin and Metastasis	Investigating the role of leptin in cancer metastasis and exploring its potential as a target for preventing the spread of cancer cells to other organs.
Preclinical Models	Utilizing advanced preclinical models, such as genetically engineered mice and organoid cultures, to better understand the complexities of leptin's role in cancer and to test potential therapies.
Cancer Microenvironment	Studying the influence of leptin on the tumor microenvironment and how it affects tumor-stroma interactions, angiogenesis, and immune responses.

A recent cell culture study revealed the effects of increasing leptin concentration on cell viability in OVCAR-3 and MDAH-2774 ovarian cancer lines using the MTT assay. Changes in the expression levels of 80 cytokines were evaluated after leptin treatment via a human cytokine antibody array. Leptin was found to increase the proliferation of both ovarian cancer cell lines. Additionally, alterations in cytokine expressions were observed in response to leptin treatment in ovarian cancer cells. These results indicated a potential role for leptin in ovarian cancer cell growth and cytokine regulation. Further research may help elucidate the implications of leptin in ovarian cancer development and treatment (Dincer et al., 2023).

Recent studies have suggested a relationship between a vegetarian diet and a decreased incidence of cardiovascular diseases, certain types of cancer, and obesity (Salehin et al., 2023; Fraser 2009; Clem and Barthel 2021). Analyzing the relationship between serum leptin concentrations and the type of diet, a study enrolled 143 female volunteers following vegetarian, vegan, or omnivore diets with normal body weight. Statistically significant differences in serum leptin concentrations were observed, with both vegetarians and vegans having significantly lower leptin levels compared to omnivores. These findings indicate that leptin levels are influenced not only by the amount of stored fat but also by the consumed food, highlighting the health-promoting properties of plant-based diets through their impact on circulating leptin (Gogga et al., 2022).

Future Research Directions and Applications

In recent years, compelling evidence from molecular, clinical, and epidemiological studies has illuminated the correlation between high plasma levels of leptin and obesity, establishing leptin as a crucial adipocytokine in mediating the molecular effects of obesity on cancer. The dysregulation of leptin has been found to impact various stages of carcinogenesis, ranging from cancer initiation and growth to metastatic progression. Moreover, researches have unveiled that leptin not only activates its canonical signaling but also interacts functionally with multiple oncogenic pathways, creating a "hyperactive leptin-signaling network" within cancer cells. This network leads to the simultaneous activation of numerous oncogenic pathways, resulting in increased proliferation, reduced apoptosis, acquiring a mesenchymal phenotype, and enhanced migration and invasion potential of tumor cells. Furthermore, leptin's influence extends beyond its canonical signaling, as it interacts with other critical molecular effectors such as estrogen, IGF-1, insulin, VEGF, and inflammatory cytokines, exerting a far-reaching impact across various tumor types. Developing a deeper understanding of the leptin-signaling network has unveiled multiple therapeutic opportunities to target crucial nodes within this network, presenting potential avenues for inhibiting leptin signaling in cancer. The basic methods and applications that can be applied for the control of leptin levels and the treatment of various cancer types can be suggested as follows on the basis of literature studies (Table 2). Considering the nutritive perspective, these findings underscore the importance of maintaining a healthy body weight and lifestyle to regulate leptin levels and mitigate its potentially adverse effects on cancer progression.

Conclusion

Proper nutrition, physical activity, and weight management are pivotal in modulating leptin secretion and sensitivity, potentially reducing the risk of cancer development and progression. As researchers delve further into the complex interplay between leptin, obesity, and cancer, nutritional interventions may emerge as complementary approaches to conventional cancer therapies. Future studies should explore how specific diets, dietary components, and lifestyle modifications can modulate leptin signaling and contribute to a favorable cancer outcome. By integrating nutritional strategies with targeted therapies to inhibit the hyperactive leptin-signaling network, we can foster a comprehensive and personalized approach to cancer prevention and treatment, ultimately leading to improved patient outcomes and better management of this challenging disease.

Disclaimer

None.

References

Bahmannia, Mahsa, Maryam Azizzade, Sahar Heydari, Javad Nasrollahzadeh, Samira Rabiei, Farah Naja, Zahra Sheikhi Mobarakeh, Jalal Hejazi, and Ehsan Hejazi. 2022. "Effects of Decaffeinated Green Coffee Extract Supplementation on Anthropometric

Indices, Blood Glucose, Leptin, Adiponectin and Neuropeptide Y (NPY) in Breast Cancer Survivors: A Randomized Clinical Trial." *Food & Function* 13 (19): 10347–56. https://doi.org/10.1039/D2FO00983H.

Bahrami, Mina, Makan Cheraghpour, Sima Jafarirad, Pejman Alavinejad, Fariba Asadi, Azita Hekmatdoost, Mahsa Mohammadi, and Zahra Yari. 2020. "The Effect of Melatonin on Treatment of Patients with Non-Alcoholic Fatty Liver Disease: A Randomized Double Blind Clinical Trial." *Complementary Therapies in Medicine* 52 (August): 102452. https://doi.org/10.1016/j.ctim.2020.102452.

Budak, Erdal, Manuel Fernández Sánchez, José Bellver, Ana Cerveró, Carlos Simón, and Antonio Pellicer. 2006. "Interactions of the Hormones Leptin, Ghrelin, Adiponectin, Resistin, and PYY3-36 with the Reproductive System." *Fertility and Sterility* 85 (6): 1563–81. https://doi.org/10.1016/j.fertnstert.2005.09.065.

Clem, Julia, and Brandon Barthel. 2021. "A Look at Plant-Based Diets." *Missouri Medicine* 118 (3): 233–38.

Dincer, Fatih, Harika Atmaca, Levent Akman, Latife Merve Oktay, Burcak Karaca, and Mustafa Cosan Terek. 2023. "Effects of Leptin on the Viability of Human Ovarian Cancer Cells and Changes in Cytokine Expression Levels." *PeerJ* 11: e15246. https://doi.org/10.7717/peerj.15246.

Dornbush, Sean, and Narothama R. Aeddula. 2023. "Physiology, Leptin." In *StatPearls*. Treasure Island (FL): StatPearls Publishing. http://www.ncbi.nlm.nih.gov/books/NBK537038/.

Du, Meizhi, Yu Wang, Jillian Vallis, Matin Shariati, Patrick S. Parfrey, John R. Mclaughlin, Peizhong Peter Wang, and Yun Zhu. 2023. "Associations between Polymorphisms in Leptin and Leptin Receptor Genes and Colorectal Cancer Survival." *Cancer Biology & Medicine* 20 (6): 438–51. https://doi.org/10.20892/j.issn.2095-3941.2022.0635.

Fraser, Gary E. 2009. "Vegetarian Diets: What Do We Know of Their Effects on Common Chronic Diseases?23." *The American Journal of Clinical Nutrition* 89 (5): 1607S-1612S. https://doi.org/10.3945/ajcn.2009.26736K.

Gencoglu, Hasan, Cemal Orhan, Mehmet Tuzcu, Nurhan Sahin, Vijaya Juturu, and Kazim Sahin. 2020. "Effects of Walnut Oil on Metabolic Profile and Transcription Factors in Rats Fed High-Carbohydrate-/-Fat Diets." *Journal of Food Biochemistry* 44 (7): e13235. https://doi.org/10.1111/jfbc.13235.

Gencoglu, Hasan. 2023. "Maca Modulates Fat and Liver Energy Metabolism Markers Insulin, IRS1, Leptin, and SIRT1 in Rats Fed Normal and High-Fat Diets." *Archives of Physiology and Biochemistry* 129 (2): 323–29. https://doi.org/10.1080/13813455.2020.1821064.

Gogga, Patrycja, Agata Janczy, Natalia Szupryczyńska, Aleksandra Śliwińska, Zdzisław Kochan, and Sylwia Malgorzewicz. 2022. "Plant-Based Diets Contribute to Lower Circulating Leptin in Healthy Subjects Independently of BMI." *Acta Biochimica Polonica* 69 (4): 879–82. https://doi.org/10.18388/abp.2020_6388.

Haidari, Fatemeh, Nasrin Banaei-Jahromi, Mehrnoosh Zakerkish, and Kambiz Ahmadi. 2020. "The Effects of Flaxseed Supplementation on Metabolic Status in Women with Polycystic Ovary Syndrome: A Randomized Open-Labeled Controlled Clinical Trial." *Nutrition Journal* 19 (1): 8. https://doi.org/10.1186/s12937-020-0524-5.

Hang, Dong, Ane Sørlie Kværner, Wenjie Ma, Yang Hu, Fred K Tabung, Hongmei Nan, Zhibin Hu, et al., 2019. "Coffee Consumption and Plasma Biomarkers of Metabolic and Inflammatory Pathways in US Health Professionals." *The American Journal of Clinical Nutrition* 109 (3): 635–47. https://doi.org/10.1093/ajcn/nqy295.

Iikuni, Noriko, Queenie Lai Kwan Lam, Liwei Lu, Giuseppe Matarese, and Antonio La Cava. 2008. "Leptin and Inflammation." *Current Immunology Reviews* 4 (2): 70–79. https://doi.org/10.2174/157339508784325046.

Klok, M. D., S. Jakobsdottir, and M. L. Drent. 2007. "The Role of Leptin and Ghrelin in the Regulation of Food Intake and Body Weight in Humans: A Review." *Obesity Reviews: An Official Journal of the International Association for the Study of Obesity* 8 (1): 21–34. https://doi.org/10.1111/j.1467-789X.2006.00270.x.

Krishnan, M. P., Sarath, Amit Gupta, Sweety Gupta, Sujata Rani, Anissa A. Mirza, and Bela Goyal. 2023. "Association of Serum Leptin With Body Mass Index in Gallbladder Cancer Patients: A Pilot Study." *Cureus* 15 (5): e39018. https://doi.org/10.7759/cureus.39018.

Ladyman, Sharon R., and David R. Grattan. 2013. "JAK-STAT and Feeding." *JAK-STAT* 2 (2): e23675. https://doi.org/10.4161/jkst.23675.

Li, Jinxia, Jingjun Xie, Xiaoqing Guo, Ruiyang Fu, Yaling Wang, and Xinjun Guan. 2023. "Effects of Mind-Regulation Acupuncture Therapy on Serum Ghrelin, Gastric Inhibitory Polypeptide, Leptin, and Insulin Levels in Breast Cancer Survivors with Cancer-Related Fatigue: A Randomized Controlled Trial." *International Journal of General Medicine* Volume 16 (March): 1017–27. https://doi.org/10.2147/IJGM.S405977.

Marttunen, Merja B., Sture Andersson, Päivi Hietanen, Sirkka-Liisa Karonen, Heikki A Koistinen, Veikko A Koivisto, Aila Tiitinen, and Olavi Ylikorkala. 2000. "Antiestrogenic Tamoxifen and Toremifene Increase Serum Leptin Levels in Postmenopausal Breast Cancer Patients." *Maturitas* 35 (2): 175–79. https://doi.org/10.1016/S0378-5122(00)00121-3.

Obradovic, Milan, Emina Sudar-Milovanovic, Sanja Soskic, Magbubah Essack, Swati Arya, Alan J. Stewart, Takashi Gojobori, and Esma R. Isenovic. 2021. "Leptin and Obesity: Role and Clinical Implication." *Frontiers in Endocrinology* 12: 585887. https://doi.org/10.3389/fendo.2021.585887.

Orhan, Cemal, Mehmet Tuzcu, Patrick Brice Deeh Defo, Nurhan Sahin, Sara Perez Ojalvo, Sarah Sylla, James R. Komorowski, and Kazim Sahin. 2022. "Effects of a Novel Magnesium Complex on Metabolic and Cognitive Functions and the Expression of Synapse-Associated Proteins in Rats Fed a High-Fat Diet." *Biological Trace Element Research* 200 (1): 247–60. https://doi.org/10.1007/s12011-021-02619-z.

Pandit, Parth, Chaitanya Shirke, Nirav Bhatia, Angel Godad, Sateesh Belemkar, Jayshree Patel, and Sandip Zine. 2023. "An Overview of Recent Findings That Shed Light on the Connection between Fat and Cancer." *Endocrine, Metabolic & Immune Disorders Drug Targets*, July. https://doi.org/10.2174/1871530323666230724141942.

Park, Hyeong-Kyu, and Rexford S. Ahima. 2015. "Physiology of Leptin: Energy Homeostasis, Neuroendocrine Function and Metabolism." *Metabolism: Clinical and Experimental* 64 (1): 24–34. https://doi.org/10.1016/j.metabol.2014.08.004.

Peng, Wei-Zhao, Xin Liu, Chao-Feng Li, and Jin Zhao. 2023. "Genetic Alterations in LEP and ADIPOQ Genes and Risk for Breast Cancer: A Meta-Analysis." *Frontiers in Oncology* 13: 1125189. https://doi.org/10.3389/fonc.2023.1125189.

Picó, Catalina, Mariona Palou, Catalina Amadora Pomar, Ana María Rodríguez, and Andreu Palou. 2022. "Leptin as a Key Regulator of the Adipose Organ." *Reviews in Endocrine & Metabolic Disorders* 23 (1): 13–30. https://doi.org/10.1007/s11154-021-09687-5.

Rashid, Aafia, Mohd Ashraf Ganie, Imtiyaz Ahmad Wani, Gulzar Ahmad Bhat, Feroz Shaheen, Ishfaq Ahmed Wani, Mukesh Shrivastava, and Zaffar Amin Shah. 2020. "Differential Impact of Insulin Sensitizers vs. Anti-Androgen on SerumLeptin Levels in Vitamin D Replete PCOS Women: A Six Month Open LabeledRandomized Study." *Hormone and Metabolic Research* 52 (02): 89–94. https://doi.org/10.1055/a-1084-5441.

Ray, Amitabha, and Margot P. Cleary. 2017. "The Potential Role of Leptin in Tumor Invasion and Metastasis." *Cytokine & Growth Factor Reviews* 38 (December): 80–97. https://doi.org/10.1016/j.cytogfr.2017.11.002.

Rosenbaum, Michael, and Rudolph L Leibel. 2014. "Role of Leptin in Energy Homeostasis in Humans." *The Journal of Endocrinology* 223 (1): T83–96. https://doi.org/10.1530/JOE-14-0358.

Salehin, Salman, Peter Rasmussen, Steven Mai, Muhammad Mushtaq, Mayank Agarwal, Syed Mustajab Hasan, Shahran Salehin, Muhammad Raja, Syed Gilani, and Wissam I. Khalife. 2023. "Plant Based Diet and Its Effect on Cardiovascular Disease." *International Journal of Environmental Research and Public Health* 20 (4): 3337. https://doi.org/10.3390/ijerph20043337.

Sánchez-Jiménez, Flora, Antonio Pérez-Pérez, Luis de la Cruz-Merino, and Víctor Sánchez-Margalet. 2019. "Obesity and Breast Cancer: Role of Leptin." *Frontiers in Oncology* 9 (July): 596. https://doi.org/10.3389/fonc.2019.00596.

Sanikini, Harinakshi, Carine Biessy, Sabina Rinaldi, Anne-Sophie Navionis, Audrey Gicquiau, Pekka Keski-Rahkonen, Agneta Kiss, et al., 2023. "Circulating Hormones and Risk of Gastric Cancer by Subsite in Three Cohort Studies." *Gastric Cancer: Official Journal of the International Gastric Cancer Association and the Japanese Gastric Cancer Association*, July. https://doi.org/10.1007/s10120-023-01414-0.

Savova, Martina S., Liliya V. Mihaylova, Daniel Tews, Martin Wabitsch, and Milen I. Georgiev. 2023. "Targeting PI3K/AKT Signaling Pathway in Obesity." *Biomedicine & Pharmacotherapy* 159 (March): 114244. https://doi.org/10.1016/j.biopha.2023.114244.

Şener, Kübra, Elif Naz Alver, and Şule Coşkun Cevher. 2022. "An Overview of Appetite Regulation Mechanisms." *Kocaeli Journal of Science and Engineering* 5 (2): 178–93. https://doi.org/10.34088/kojose.1091078.

Słomian, Grzegorz, Elżbieta Świętochowska, Grzegorz Nowak, Krystyna Pawlas, Aleksandra Żelazko, and Przemysław Nowak. 2017. "Chemotherapy and Plasma Adipokines Level in Patients with Colorectal Cancer." *Postepy Higieny I Medycyny Doswiadczalnej* (Online) 71 (0): 281–90. https://doi.org/10.5604/01.3001.0010.3813.

Stępień, Sebastian, Paweł Olczyk, Joanna Gola, Katarzyna Komosińska-Vassev, and Aleksandra Mielczarek-Palacz. 2023. "The Role of Selected Adipocytokines in Ovarian Cancer and Endometrial Cancer." *Cells* 12 (8): 1118. https://doi.org/10.3390/cells12081118.

Sturgeon, Kathleen, Laura Digiovanni, Jerene Good, Domenick Salvatore, Desiré Fenderson, Susan Domchek, Jill Stopfer, et al., 2016. "Exercise-Induced Dose-Response Alterations in Adiponectin and Leptin Levels Are Dependent on Body Fat Changes in Women at Risk for Breast Cancer." *Cancer Epidemiology, Biomarkers & Prevention* 25 (8): 1195–1200. https://doi.org/10.1158/1055-9965.EPI-15-1087.

Varela, Luis, and Tamas L Horvath. 2012. "Leptin and Insulin Pathways in POMC and AgRP Neurons That Modulate Energy Balance and Glucose Homeostasis." *EMBO Reports* 13 (12): 1079–86. https://doi.org/10.1038/embor.2012.174.

Zhao, Shangang, Christine M. Kusminski, Joel K. Elmquist, and Philipp E. Scherer. 2020. "Leptin: Less Is More." *Diabetes* 69 (5): 823–29. https://doi.org/10.2337/dbi19-0018.

Zhou, Xueqing, Shuya Yang, Qianqian Liu, Ran Wei, Jing Liu, Naixiang Luo, and Wenhui Liu. 2022. "[Leptin promotes the proliferation and migration of MDA-MB-231 breast cancer cells by up regulating MMP14]." Xi Bao Yu Fen Zi Mian Yi Xue Za Zhi = *Chinese Journal of Cellular and Molecular Immunology* 38 (1): 39–47.

Chapter 7

A Molecular Overview of Leptin in Several Pathological Conditions

Muge Atis Ceylan[*] and Hilal Eren Gozel

Department of Medical Biology and Genetics,
Istanbul Okan University School of Medicine, Istanbul, Türkey

Abstract

Leptin is a 16 kDa peptide hormone that is the product of *LEP* (also known as *OB*) gene. The Leptin gene is primarily expressed in white adipocytes. Although the leptin hormone is mainly associated with the regulation of body weight and energy expenditure via hypothalamic leptin receptors, it has a diverse range of effects on different physiological functions such as inflammatory responses, hematopoiesis, angiogenesis, reproduction, bone formation, and wound healing. Besides having pleiotropic effects on metabolism, dysfunction of the leptin gene family and its cognate receptor, leptin receptor (LR), may result in pathological conditions for several diseases including obesity, cardiovascular diseases, infertility, and inflammation.

Pathophysiological manifestations of these diseases indicate the important role of leptin signaling. In the present chapter, we reviewed variations in gene expressions of the leptin gene family and LR, along with the role of leptin in insulin resistance, immunotherapy, tumor progression, and inflammation. In this concept, the chapter covers molecular overview for selected diseases, leptin sensitivity at the cellular level, and epigenetic regulations involving the expression of the leptin gene. Finally, the potential of leptin was discussed as a candidate

---

[*] Corresponding Author's Email: muge.atis@okan.edu.tr.

In: Leptin and its Role in Health and Disease
Editor: Stephen E. Bradley
ISBN: 979-8-89113-274-0
© 2024 Nova Science Publishers, Inc.

biomarker and a new immunotherapy approach for the treatment. Our objective provides a comprehensive review on the importance of leptin during different pathological conditions.

Keywords: leptin, diseases, molecular mechanism, obesity, insulin

Introduction

Leptin (from the Greek leptos=thin) hormone was first described in 1994 (Zhang et al. 1994). It functions as a satiety factor and has a direct role in the homeostatic regulation of body weight. It is a 16 kDa peptide hormone that is encoded in *LEP* (also known as *OB*) gene (Trayhurn et al. 1999).

Leptin is a part of the adipocytokine signaling pathway. The principle of leptin production mainly correlates with increased adipocyte density. As a regulator, leptin regulates the energy intake and metabolic rate of organisms at hypothalamic nuclei in the central nervous system. Its anorectic effects are manifested by modulating the levels of neuropeptides such as Neuropeptide Y, α-Melanocyte-stimulating hormone, and Agouti-related protein. In addition, a class of proteins like adaptor proteins works for appropriate cellular response. Namely, adaptor proteins connect related proteins which further initiates the signaling cascade. The signaling pathway of leptin acts through receptor tyrosine kinases or receptor-associated tyrosine kinases (e.g., Janus kinases (JAKs)). Specifically, in the JAKs activation, phosphorylation of the receptors and associated kinases serve as a binding site for adaptor proteins that have phosphotyrosine-binding motifs, Src homology 2 (SH2) or phosphotyrosine binding (PTB) domains (Maures, Kurzer, and Carter-Su 2007). Those adaptor proteins have typical modular structures that link multiple proteins. The adaptation ability of those proteins makes it possible to respond particularly in a diverse environment (Maures, Kurzer, and Carter-Su 2007).

While leptin is transferred by the leptin receptor (LR) from extracellular fluid to intracellular fluid, the cascade influences a variety of signaling pathways including mitogen-activated protein kinase (MAPK), AMP-activated protein kinase (AMPK), STAT cascade, and, PI3K pathway. However, the Jak/STAT pathway is the main signaling mechanism during leptin receptor activation (Huo and Luo 2011). The leptin receptor is a single membrane-spanning receptor under the class 1 cytokine receptor family (Tartaglia et al. 1995). The variety of LR is counted from LRa to LRd for murine as well as the three human LR isoforms are present (Kloek et al. 2002). Human and murine variants of the receptor share the same complex extracellular domain, which consists of two cytokine receptor homology (CRH) domains separated by immunoglobulin (Ig)-like domain and followed by two membrane-proximal fibronectin type III (FN III) domains (Tartaglia et al. 1995). Leptin receptor isoforms have three forms: secreted, short, and long. The secreted forms are the products of alternative splicing (e.g., murine LRe) or proteolytic cleavage of membrane-bound LR forms (Ge et al. 2002). Additionally, there are murine LRa, LRc, and LRd short forms of leptin receptors but their physiological functions still do not be understood well. Leptin receptor-b (LRb) is highly conserved during evolutionary stages (Kloek et al. 2002). Besides the unknown function of short LR forms, LRb is critical for the leptin signaling pathway. This form has a long cytoplasmic region containing a variety of motifs for leptin activation. The other forms partially have or lack all of these motifs. This situation makes the LRb isoform the most studied one among all other isoforms for leptin signaling (Friedman and Halaas 1998). Leptin receptor-b contains a 282-amino acid extension (total 301-amino acid intracellular tail) to activate intracellular signaling. Activation of signaling pathways vigorously starts upon leptin binding. Also, it was shown that Jak2 is the only Jak kinase activated during phosphorylation and required for the LRb signaling. Additionally, some of the LRb sequences are essential for Jak2 tyrosine phosphorylation. The sequences of the LR isoforms are diverse, and none of the other forms of LR, rather than LRb, mediate the activation of Jak2 at physiologic levels (Kloek et al. 2002). Leptin receptor b activation also induces phosphorylation of various members of the insulin receptor substrate (IRS) family, including IRS1 and particularly IRS2. The complex pathway needs an adaptor protein SH2B1. The binding of SH2B1 to Jak2 facilitated leptin-dependent pathways of Jak2. As far as we know, Jak2 was required for leptin-stimulated phosphorylation of IRS1, an upstream activator of the phosphatidylinositol 3-kinase pathway (PI3K) (Li et al. 2007). In addition to leptin as a hormone, insulin is also accounted as a main regulator in the hypothalamic region for energy metabolism and food intake in the central nervous system. The relationship between leptin and insulin via the PI3K pathway in energy homeostasis was demonstrated *in vivo* and *in vitro* studies (Mirshamsi et al. 2004; Benomar et al. 2005). The relative coordination of insulin and leptin in the function of energy metabolism is difficult to address; however, the role of the PI3K pathway is essential (Wauman and Tavernier 2011).

Many organs participating in lipid metabolism are mostly under the control of the leptin hormone. As an adipose-derived hormone, leptin has profound effects on energy homeostasis and storage in the brain. It acts directly on the hypothalamic neurons of the central nervous system. Modulation of appetite and energy balance is controlled by leptin-responsive neurons including AgRP and POMC neurons. Those leptin-responsive neurons are interconnected with the other cells of the brain via LRb, the long form of leptin receptor in the hypothalamus. This neurocircuit is activated by the anorexigenic action of LRb activating Jak2- dependent and Jak2-independent pathways. Those pathways are associated with STAT3, PI 3-kinase, MAPK, AMPK, and mTOR cascade. Negative (SOCS3, PTP1B) and positive (SH2B1) regulators manage the energy demand of the neurocircuit (Morris and Rui 2009). One of the *in vivo* studies stated that leptin increases glucose uptake and fatty acid oxidation in skeletal muscle. An increase in glucose uptake in skeletal muscle is associated with leptin via the hypothalamic–sympathetic nervous system axis and β-adrenergic mechanism. Also, leptin stimulates fatty acid oxidation in muscle via AMPK (Minokoshi, Toda, and Okamoto 2012). In addition, leptin regulates the activation of hepatic AMPK through the central nervous system and α-adrenergic sympathetic nerves in the liver (Miyatomo et al. 2012).

Another leptin-induced pathway is related to the STAT cascade. *In vitro* studies demonstrated that upon binding of leptin to its receptor, there are activations of STAT1, STAT3, and STAT5 (Friedmann and Halaas 1998). Whereas *in vivo* studies showed that leptin activates only the STAT3 cascade. Vaisse and colleagues investigated that the direct target of leptin in the hypothalamus and gp-130-like leptin receptors play a crucial role in the activation of STAT3. The STAT cascade starts with the binding of the STAT proteins to phosphotyrosine residues in the cytoplasmic domain of the ligand-activated receptor where they are phosphorylated. The dimerization of activated STAT proteins is translocated to the nucleus where they bind DNA and regulate transcription. It was known that in a variety of mouse tissues known to express LR; however, hormone-induced STAT activation was constrained to the localized region in the brain (Vaisse et al. 1996).

Epigenetics of Leptin

Lipid metabolism also seems to be regulated epigenetically. A study conducted on overweight and obese people revealed that hypermethylation of

DNA is associated with lipid metabolism. There is a list of certain genes that regulate cholesterol metabolism and hypermethylation of CpG loci located in promoters of genes. Those genes are *LRP1, ABCG1, PCSK9, SREBF1, ANGPTL4*, and *NR1H2* in hypercholesterolemic patients. Novel epigenetically regulated CpG sites also include *ABCG4, AP2A2, ANGPTL4, AP2M1, CLTC, FGF19, AP2S1, FGF1R, HDLBP, LMF1, LIPA, LRP5, LSR, ZDHHC8* and *NR1H2* genes. As a result, Platek and colleagues suggested that obese individuals with hypercholesterolemia possess a certain DNA methylation pattern that affects lipid metabolism (Platek et al. 2020). Moreover, imprinting as an epigenetic regulation also contributes to the activity of the leptin gene. Allard et al. stated that in some metabolic diseases such as obesity and type-2 diabetes, epigenetic regulation of leptin genes plays a role. They showed that maternal glycemia during pregnancy influences the trajectory of offspring's metabolic activity after birth (Allard et al. 2015).

Leptin as a Feedback System

Many physiological systems use feedback mechanisms to balance energy metabolism. Likewise, leptin levels in circulation act as a feedback system. The main physiologic role of leptin is to create a balance between appetite and energy expenditure. The reduced ability of leptin promotes the risk factor for obesity. In that sense, the term "leptin resistance" is used to address the reduced ability of the leptin hormone. Increased levels of circulating leptin seem to be a paradox for obese individuals. One of the underlying mechanisms for this phenomenon is stated as defective leptin transport (Wauman and Tavernier 2011). Relative or total insensitivity for leptin binding regions mostly resulted in obesity. An increase in circulating leptin is a kind of mimicry of increased insulin levels observed in insulin-resistant diabetes.

High leptin concentration in the bloodstream can upregulate the methionine adenosyltransferase (MAT) enzyme that catalyzes a methyl donor, S-adenosylmethionine; which increases the expression of MAT2A that promotes hepatic stellate cell (HSC) activity. It was known that liver fibrogenesis originated from HSC activation in obese people. A direct effect of MAT2A activity on liver fibrosis was shown as a result of leptin-induced HSC. Hyperleptinaemia conditions can be related to the β-catenin pathway, and a decrease in the expression of one of the transcription factors, E2F-4. E2F-4 could bind to MAT2A promoter which inhibits MAT2A promoter activity. Therefore, MAT2 expression in HSC is promoted by leptin via the β-catenin pathway in response to the downregulation of E2F-4 (Cheng et al. 2020).

Table 1. A summary of Dysfunction of leptin and diseases include more than one mechanism including specific regulators for obesity in elderly and infants

Regulation of Lipid Metabolism	Mechanisms	Specific Regulators	References
Obesity	Hypermethylation of DNA	CpG loci of *LRP1, ABCG1, PCSK9, SREBF1, ANGPTL4, NR1H2*	Platek et al. 2020
Obesity	Enzyme activity plus transcription factor	Methionine adenosyltransferase activity under the regulation of E2F-4	Cheng et al. 2020
Obesity	Epigenetic regulation	Maternal Glycemia	Allard et al. 2015
Obesity in offspring	mRNA expression	mRNA level of the leptin gene	Lecoutre et al. 2016
Hypertension	Gene conversion	Microsatellite polymorphism	Akhter et al. 2012
Non-alcoholic fatty liver diseases	Hormonal	Leptin level in blood	Marques et al. 2021

In one of the studies, a low level of leptin in serum is correlated with functional hypothalamic amenorrhea (FHA). Altered nutritional conditions and eating patterns of women with FHA can result in lower leptin parallel with thyroid levels. The study stated low leptin resulted from the condition metabolic/nutritional insult in those women (Warren et al. 1999).

As well as leptin, LR and molecular components of signaling pathways promote the pathophysiology of obesity, also gender and psychological factors contribute to the differences in leptin production and leptin sensitivity (Wauman and Tavernier 2011; Hellstrom et al. 2000; Friedman 2002). In developmental stages, the maternal genomic state can also affect the offspring. One of the studies examined gonadal and perirenal fat pads to evaluate metabolic programming induced by maternal obesity. Lecoutre et al. stated there is a significant increase in the mRNA expression level of leptin in newborns. In addition, maternal obesity did affect LRb (Lecoutre et al. 2016). As a result of changes in gene expression and hormonal levels of leptin, many metabolic diseases including obesity, hypertension, and non-alcoholic fatty liver can be observed (Table 1).

Homeostasis keeps the physiological system stable and sustainable. Any disruption can result in dysregulation of lipid metabolism. Underlying mechanisms for the pathology of diseases such as obesity in the elderly and infants, hypertension, and non-alcoholic fatty liver disease summarize the disruption of lipid metabolism regulation due to genetic, hormonal, and epigenetic factors. Some of the diseases are directly linked with lipid metabolism regulation. In literature, obesity in offspring is related to the expression of maternal mRNA level of leptin. Also, leptin hormone level is associated with non-alcoholic fatty liver diseases. The underlying mechanism of hypertension is shown as gene conversion regulations of the leptin gene. Lastly, changes in hypermethylation of DNA, enzyme activity, and epigenetic regulations are the main reasons for obesity (Table 1). Variations of the leptin gene family and its receptor may affect an array of diseases. In literature, most of the studies focused on the role of leptin in obesity; however, cancer and infertility have been on the radar of leptin-related diseases for over 20 years (Table 2).

Table 2. Regulation of leptin and its receptor is associated with other certain genes in cancer and infertility

Diseases	Mechanisms	Specific Regulators	References
Breast Cancer	Overexpression of genes	Leptin plus ADIPOQ genes	Cedano-Prieto et al. 2022
Osteosarcoma, Breast Cancer	Overexpression of genes	OCT3/4, Nanog, Sox2 and Leptin	Paino et al. 2017
Hepatocellular Carcinoma	Leptin Signaling	Wild type Leptin gene in zebrafish	Yang et al. 2019
Infertility	Receptor Expression	LepR	Ishikawa et al. 2007

Leptin and Diseases

Leptin seems to be related to a wide variety of diseases including cancer, cardiovascular problems, infertility, rare diseases, and many more. Having a crucial role in balancing energy expenditure and body weight, it is quite logical that if this metabolism disrupts, it may cause several problems in the body. However, in the literature there are conflicting results about the main reason for these diseases is leptin or weight gain, or both.

Cancer and Leptin

Many studies suggest that leptin dysregulation may lead to varied cancer types. *ADIPOQ* gene is known for energy metabolism which is related to cancer progression. Especially in breast cancer, other genes such as *OCT3/4, Nanog*, and *Sox2* contribute to the pathogenesis of breast cancer as well as other cancer types like osteosarcoma. Researchers studied survivin gene, a molecular biomarker in cancer, and survivin variants of breast cancer are relieved that adipokines *LEP* expression changes due to different stages of cancer. Therefore, they suggested that *LEP* can be assigned as a biomarker.

In the highlighted study, it was known that *LEP* overexpression in early stages of breast cancer (IA and IIA) is observed and there is a subsequent decrease in more advanced stages. Furthermore, this study reveals S-2B as an interesting variant of breast cancer. First, in the study, S-2B and its wild-type variant, S-WT, relate the correlation between *LEP* and *ADIPOQ* genes (Cedano-Prieto et al. 2022). In another study, Piano and colleagues investigated the potentials of cancer cells on human adipose stem cells differentiation, and they found upregulation of cohorts of genes including OCT3/4, Nanog, Sox2, and leptin in which co-cultured either SAOS2 osteosarcoma or MCF7 breast cancer cells with human adipose stem cells (hASCs). They observed that both SAOS2 and MCF7 cell lines induced an increase in hASCs proliferation (Paino et al. 2017).

Also, studies on animal models showed that cancer-associated muscle wasting can be associated with blocking leptin signaling activation (Yang et al. 2019). In another study, researchers used zebrafish as a model organism to investigate the effect of leptin signaling in hepatocellular carcinoma. Finally, different research groups reported a partial role of leptin in immunotherapy, tumor progression, and also some rare diseases (Zhang et al. 2018; Allard et al. 2015; Wang et al. 2019).

Cardiovascular Diseases (CVD) and Leptin

Emerging evidence from both animal and human studies indicate that there may be a correlation between leptin and cardiovascular diseases associated with obesity. Moreover; high leptin levels may be linked to cardiovascular complications along with hypertension, diabetes, coronary heart disease, and stroke (Huo and Luo 2011). Some rat studies demonstrate that the injection of leptin increases blood pressure (Correia and Haynes 2004).

Nalini and colleagues worked on human blood samples from normal-weight, overweight, and obese patients with a history of cardiovascular diseases (CVD). They found a positive correlation between leptin and body mass index subjects in both CVD and control subjects (Nalini et al. 2015).

It was also known that gene conversion mechanisms are also important when we consider the occurrence of diseases. One study showed that leptin gene variation on 3' flanking regions showed a significant association of microsatellite polymorphism with hypertension patients with high body mass index; however, there was a slight association with hypertension patients with low body mass. They concluded that genetic variations in the 3' flanking region of leptin genes significantly affect hypertensive conditions (Akhter et al. 2012).

Infertility and Leptin

The metabolic activities of cells involve many mechanisms. One of the most critical metabolic activities is cellular division as leptin participates in energy balance, and dysfunctions of cellular activity result in various types of diseases.

Leptin plays an important role in sexual development and fertility. Studies show that *ob* gene knockout male and female mice are infertile. Remarkably, when treated with leptin, female ob/ob mice become pregnant and deliver (Chehab, Lim, and Lu 1996; Kiess, Blum, and Aubert 1998). On the contrary, researchers also showed that infertility may be related to the hyper-function of leptin. Excessive leptin levels negatively affect sperm parameters of individuals with high-fat percentages or BMI (Malik, Durairajanayagam, and Singh 2019). One of the studies showed an increase in the expression of leptin and its receptor was associated with infertility in men. The study focused on the relationship between the expression of leptin, leptin receptor in the testis and spermatogenesis, and testosterone (T) concentration in infertile men. Immunostaining of LR showed that primarily in Leydig cells, leptin receptor expression of Leydig cells was inversely correlated with serum T concentration. This study stated the dysfunction of spermatogenesis is associated with an increase in leptin and its receptor expression in the testis (Ishikawa et al. 2007).

In pregnancy, leptin has additional roles such as implantation and formation of blastocyst. Fetal leptin assists placental angiogenesis, induces placental growth, and protects the fetus from the maternal immune system. When this elaborate molecule has some dysfunction, it may cause problems in pregnancy. When compared to normal pregnancy, serum leptin levels increase in pre-eclamptic pregnancy (Jaiswar and Priyadarshini 2021). Regulation of female pubertal development via leptin is more pronounced when compared to male pubertal development since low levels of leptin are sufficient for males (Vázquez, Romero-Ruiz, and Tena-Sempere 2015). For female infertility, high serum leptin levels are correlated to patients with polycystic ovary syndrome (PCOS) (Chen et al. 2013). Moreover, long-term galactosemia can result in Primary Ovarian Insufficiency (POI). And it is reported that there is a dysregulation of the expression of *LEP* and LEPR in classical galactosemia regardless of gender (Colhoun et al. 2018).

Rare Diseases and Leptin

Metabolic syndromes affect the primary regulation of homeostasis, and multiple defects of different organs cause severe results. In the case of rare diseases, various physiological systems predominantly suffer from dysregulation of the immune system. In this section, we consider the role of leptin which has a correlation with immune disorders, and insulin resistance in the case of rare diseases. Leptin hormone levels in blood plasma are the main focus for one of the rare diseases like Acquired Generalized Lipodystrophy (AGL). The characteristics of the disease are a rare immune-mediated disorder with adipose tissue loss and its complications related to insulin resistance mechanisms. Alexandre and colleagues reported that a patient with metastatic melanoma having the implications of rapid loss of subcutaneous adipose tissue and diabetes was diagnosed as having severe insulin resistance and more importantly lack of leptin in plasma. In AGL, the role of leptin may be regulating innate and adaptive immunity. In this case study report, they concluded a risk-benefit ratio for leptin replacement therapy should be considered during advanced cancer therapy (Jehl et al. 2019).

Another disease called familial partial lipodystrophy (FPLD) is characterized by partial loss of subcutaneous fat. Most common types as FPLD types 2 and 3. Those are variants associated with specific genes. These are *LMNA* (FPLD type 2 or Dunnigan, OMIM number: #151660, dominant) and *PPARG* (FPLD type 3, OMIM number: #604367, dominant) genes (Peters et al. 1998; Barroso et al. 1999). Variants within *LMNA* and *PPARG* genes were responsible for more than 50% of all reported FPLD patients. Heterogeneity and rarity of FPLD cases easily misdiagnosed. Therefore, the genetic background of FPLD needs to be sequenced for *LMNA* and *PPARG* genes (Rutkowska et al. 2022). It was reported that *LMNA* and *PPARG* cause insulin resistance. It was reported that leptin levels in *LMNA* pathogenic variants were higher compared with *PPARG* (Akinci et al. 2017). Furthermore, Bardet-Biedl syndrome (BBS) is another rare genetic disorder and the phenotype of the disease stands for neuroendocrine origin. Büscher stated a significant increase in leptin levels in the plasma of patients with BBS (Buscher et al. 2012).

Leptin as a Biomarker and a Possible Candidate for Treatment Options

Leptin level is mostly measured from blood plasma and that is the direct way of monitoring the circulating leptin level. This situation makes leptin a useful candidate for disease biomarkers. Scientists reported that leptin was one of the circulating biomarkers for chronic liver conditions such as nonalcoholic fatty liver diseases (Marques et al. 2021).

In a recent study, leptin was considered a new immunotherapy approach. Wang and colleagues investigated immunotherapy over obesity. They emphasized immune regulation changes as a result of obesity and stated that PD-(L)-1 mediated T cell dysfunction is partially driven by leptin. Their data showed a direct interaction between increased PD-1 expression and upregulation of phospho-STAT3 (pSTAT3) which is a downstream mediator of leptin signaling. Therefore, the cascade causes the induction of PD-1 expression in T cells, ultimately. They also examined the inhibition of pSTAT3 in that context, and this resulted in decreased activity of upregulated pSTAT3 and PD-1 driven by leptin. In this scenario, leptin was a bridge between obesity and PD-1 expression. Then, they examined the effects of leptin on T-cell exhaustion in tumor-bearing models using leptin-deficient mice and recombinant mouse leptin. They suggested that tumor growth and immune activity were affected by leptin signaling. Leptin signaling interacts with promoting T cell exhaustion in tumor-bearing mice. Therefore, they proposed that the link between leptin and immunotherapy can be a new approach for PD-1 and T cell dysfunction in cancer progression. (Wang et al. 2019).

Leptin and Treatment

Today's technology offers a wide choice of treatment options. Especially, defining new roles of microRNAs opens up new opportunities for treatment. For this purpose, we listed miRNA which directly or indirectly participated in the regulation of leptin gene expression.

Immunotherapy is another option for the treatment of leptin-causing diseases due to increased inflammatory cytokines such as TNF-α, IL-6 as observed in many diseases like nonalcoholic fatty liver disease (NAFLD)(Dongiovanni et al. 2018). The role of AdipoR2, a receptor for adiponectin, in lipid and glucose metabolism, through enhancing the activity of the PPARα pathway, both ameliorating insulin resistance and steatosis, is also associated with NAFLD. One of the studies showed that AdipoR2 was the target of miR-375 in HepG2 cells and a reduction of AdipoR2 level was observed in high fat diet-induced NAFLD mice. In this study, both the mRNA level and the protein expression level of AdipoR2 were reduced in HepG2 cells during overexpression of miR-375. In addition, the inhibition of mirR-375 was reversed by silencing AdipoR2 in PA-induced HepG2 cells, and there was a reduced activity of TNF-α, IL-6 as well as leptin and the production of adiponectin. As a result, this study demonstrated that AdipoR2 is a direct target of miR-375 and that up-regulation of AdipoR2 by miR-375 may play a role in NAFLD (Lei et al. 2018). For the first time, the study documented changes in hypothalamic miRNA expression profiles of various nutritional challenges. They conducted experiments on male rats who are under extreme nutritional stress, namely chronic caloric restriction and high-fat diet–induced obesity conditions. Analyses allowed the identification of sets of miRNAs, including let-7a, mir-132, mir-145, mir-9*, mir-218, and mir-30e whose expression patterns in the hypothalamus were changed by fasting conditions (Sangiao-Alvarellos et al. 2014). They stated that there was an increase in let-7a, mir-132, mir-145, and mir-9* miRNA expression levels in the hypothalamus which were caused by fasting, and the effect was completely reversed by treatment with leptin. According to results for leptin treatment of the fed *ad libitum* group, there was an increase in miRNA expression levels for mir-218 and mir-30e which was reported as opposite results in rats subjected to fasting (Sangiao-Alvarellos et al. 2014). Hypothalamic control is essential to regulate energy homeostasis and the role of leptin is always in the center of obesity-related studies. Therefore, these studies provide potential tools to use miRNA regulatory pathways as a possible target for the treatment of obesity, inflammation, and neurodegenerative diseases.

Conclusion

Leptin is mostly associated with obesity and related diseases like hypertension and cardiovascular diseases (Tables 1 and 2). Moreover, differences in the expression of leptin and LR can be a causative factor for cardiovascular diseases, cancer, infertility, and rare diseases. One can ask why the dysfunction of leptin has such a large-scale effect on varied diseases. The answer is not clear, however, we know that the roles of leptin in energy homeostasis provide a quite large system to interfere. As fluctuations of hormone levels in plasma or changes in the expression of LR influence the actions of leptin and this gives a huge ability to leptin that these effects can be observed from the central nervous system through the immune system. We should also note that *in vivo* and *in vitro* studies provide controversial results about the increase or decrease of leptin or LR-causing diseases.

Do obesity-related pathologies cause diseases due to dysfunction of leptin or dysfunction of leptin because of secondary pathologies related to other metabolic syndromes? The task is quite challenging to answer. Because complex interactions for leptin level in plasma and the role of LR targets different signaling pathways in a synergic or antagonist manner.

Therefore, leptin signaling in pathological cases has yet undiscovered targets for treatments; however, as the last two parts of the chapter indicated, leptin is an effective candidate for biomarker if the signaling pathway is well defined and with the help of emerging miRNA technologies, immunotherapy can be an option for the treatment of leptin-causing diseases.

References

Akhter, Q., A. Masood, R. Ashraf, S. Majid, S. Rasool, T. Khan, T. Rashid, A. S. Sameer, and B. A. Ganai. "Polymorphisms in the 3' Utr of the Human Leptin Gene and Their Role in Hypertension." [In English]. *Molecular Medicine Reports* 5, no. 4 (Apr 2012): 1058-62.

Akinci, B., H. Onay, T. Demir, S. Savas-Erdeve, R. Gen, I. Y. Simsir, F. E. Keskin, Erturk, M. S., Uzum, A. K., Yaylali, G. F., Ozdemir, N. K., Atik, T., Ozen, S., Yurekli, B. S., Apaydin, T., Altay, C., Akinci, G., Demir, L., Comlekci, A., ... Oral, E. A. "Clinical Presentations, Metabolic Abnormalities and End-Organ Complications in Patients with Familial Partial Lipodystrophy." [In English]. *Metabolism-Clinical and Experimental* 72 (Jul 2017): 109-19.

Allard, C., V. Desgagne, J. Patenaude, M. Lacroix, L. Guillemette, M. C. Battista, M. Doyon, Ménard, J., Ardilouze, J., Perron, P., Bouchard, L., & Hivert, M. "Mendelian Randomization Supports Causality between Maternal Hyperglycemia and Epigenetic Regulation of Leptin Gene in Newborns." [In English]. *Epigenetics* 10, no. 4 (Apr 2015): 342-51.

Barroso, I., M. Gurnell, V. E. Crowley, M. Agostini, J. W. Schwabe, M. A. Soos, G. L. Maslen, Williams, T. D. M., Lewis, H., Schafer, A. J., Chatterjee, V. K. K., & O'Rahilly, S. "Dominant Negative Mutations in Human Ppargamma Associated with Severe Insulin Resistance, Diabetes Mellitus and Hypertension." *Nature* 402, no. 6764 (Dec 23-30 1999): 880-3.

Benomar, Y., A. F. Roy, A. Aubourg, J. Djiane, and M. Taouis. "Cross Down-Regulation of Leptin and Insulin Receptor Expression and Signalling in a Human Neuronal Cell Line." *Biochem J* 388, no. Pt 3 (Jun 15 2005): 929-39.

Buscher, A. K., M. Cetiner, R. Buscher, A. M. Wingen, B. P. Hauffa, and P. F. Hoyer. "Obesity in Patients with Bardet-Biedl Syndrome: Influence of Appetite-Regulating Hormones." [In English]. *Pediatric Nephrology* 27, no. 11 (Nov 2012): 2065-71.

Cedano-Prieto, D. M., F. Bergez-Hernandez, E. A. Leal-Leon, N. Garcia-Magallanes, F. Luque-Ortega, V. Picos-Cardenas, E. Guerrero-Arambula, Gutierrez-Zepeda, B., Romo-Martinez, E., & Arambula-Meraz, E. "Altered Expression of Survivin Variants S-2b and S-Wt in Breast Cancer Is Related to Adipokine Expression." *J Oncol* 2022 (2022): 7398444.

Chehab, F. E., M. E. Lim, and R. H. Lu. "Correction of the Sterility Defect in Homozygous Obese Female Mice by Treatment with the Human Recombinant Leptin." [In English]. *Nature Genetics* 12, no. 3 (Mar 1996): 318-20.

Chen, X. W., X. Jia, J. Qiao, Y. F. Guan, and J. H. Kang. "Adipokines in Reproductive Function: A Link between Obesity and Polycystic Ovary Syndrome." [In English]. *Journal of Molecular Endocrinology* 50, no. 2 (Apr 2013): R21-R37.

Cheng, F., S. Su, X. Zhu, X. Jia, H. Tian, X. Zhai, W. Guan, and Y. Zhou. "Leptin Promotes Methionine Adenosyltransferase 2a Expression in Hepatic Stellate Cells by the Downregulation of E2f-4 Via the Beta-Catenin Pathway." *FASEB J* 34, no. 4 (Apr 2020): 5578-89.

Colhoun, H. O., E. M. Rubio Gozalbo, A. M. Bosch, I. Knerr, C. Dawson, J. Brady, M. Galligan, Stepien, K., O'Flaherty, R., Catherine Moss, C., Peter Barker, P., Fitzgibbon, M., Doran, P. P., & Treacy, E. P. "Fertility in Classical Galactosaemia, a Study of N-Glycan, Hormonal and Inflammatory Gene Interactions." *Orphanet J Rare Dis* 13, no. 1 (Sep 19 2018): 164.

Correia, M. L. D., and W. G. Haynes. "Leptin, Obesity and Cardiovascular Disease." [In English]. *Current Opinion in Nephrology and Hypertension* 13, no. 2 (Mar 2004): 215-23.

Dongiovanni, P., M. Meroni, M. Longo, S. Fargion, and A. L. Fracanzani. "Mirna Signature in Nafld: A Turning Point for a Non-Invasive Diagnosis." *Int J Mol Sci* 19, no. 12 (Dec 10 2018).

Friedman, J. M. "The Function of Leptin in Nutrition, Weight, and Physiology." *Nutr Rev* 60, no. 10 Pt 2 (Oct 2002): S1-14; discussion S68-84, 85-7.

Friedman, J. M., and J. L. Halaas. "Leptin and the Regulation of Body Weight in Mammals." [In English]. *Nature* 395, no. 6704 (Oct 22 1998): 763-70.

Ge, H. F., L. Huang, T. Pourbahrami, and C. Li. "Generation of Soluble Leptin Receptor by Ectodomain Shedding of Membrane-Spanning Receptors in Vitro and in Vivo." [In English]. *Journal of Biological Chemistry* 277, no. 48 (Nov 29 2002): 45898-903.

Hellstrom, L., H. Wahrenberg, K. Hruska, S. Reynisdottir, and P. Arner. "Mechanisms Behind Gender Differences in Circulating Leptin Levels." *J Intern Med* 247, no. 4 (Apr 2000): 457-62.

Hou, N., and J. D. Luo. "Leptin and Cardiovascular Diseases." [In English]. *Clinical and Experimental Pharmacology and Physiology* 38, no. 12 (Dec 2011): 905-13.

Ishikawa, T., H. Fujioka, T. Ishimura, A. Takenaka, and M. Fujisawa. "Expression of Leptin and Leptin Receptor in the Testis of Fertile and Infertile Patients." *Andrologia* 39, no. 1 (Feb 2007): 22-7.

Jaiswar, S. P. and A. Priyadarshini. *Leptin and Female Reproductive Health.* Weight Management - Challenges and Opportunities. Edited by H. M. Heshmati. United Kingdom: IntechOpen, 2021. doi:10.5772/intechopen.95719.

Jehl, A., C. Cugnet-Anceau, C. Vigouroux, A. L. Legeay, S. Dalle, O. Harou, L. Marchand, Lascols, O., Caussy, C., Thivolet, C., Laville, M., & Disse, E. "Acquired Generalized Lipodystrophy: A New Cause of Anti-Pd-1 Immune-Related Diabetes." [In English]. *Diabetes Care* 42, no. 10 (Oct 2019): 2008-10.

Kiess, W., W. F. Blum, and M. L. Aubert. "Leptin, Puberty and Reproductive Function: Lessons from Animal Studies and Observations in Humans." [In English]. *European Journal of Endocrinology* 138, no. 1 (Jan 1998): 26-29.

Kloek, C., A. K. Haq, S. L. Dunn, H. J. Lavery, A. S. Banks, and M. G. Myers, Jr. "Regulation of Jak Kinases by Intracellular Leptin Receptor Sequences." *J Biol Chem* 277, no. 44 (Nov 1 2002): 41547-55.

Lecoutre, S., B. Deracinois, C. Laborie, D. Eberle, C. Guinez, P. E. Panchenko, J. Lesage, Vieau, D., Junien, C., Gabory, A., & Breton, C. "Depot- and Sex-Specific Effects of Maternal Obesity in Offspring's Adipose Tissue." *J Endocrinol* 230, no. 1 (Jul 2016): 39-53.

Lei, L., C. Zhou, X. Yang, and L. Li. "Down-Regulation of Microrna-375 Regulates Adipokines and Inhibits Inflammatory Cytokines by Targeting Adipor2 in Non-Alcoholic Fatty Liver Disease." *Clin Exp Pharmacol Physiol* 45, no. 8 (Aug 2018): 819-31.

Li, Z., Y. Zhou, C. Carter-Su, M. G. Myers, Jr., and L. Rui. "Sh2b1 Enhances Leptin Signaling by Both Janus Kinase 2 Tyr813 Phosphorylation-Dependent and -Independent Mechanisms." *Mol Endocrinol* 21, no. 9 (Sep 2007): 2270-81.

Malik, I. A., D. Durairajanayagam, and H. J. Singh. "Leptin and Its Actions on Reproduction in Males." [In English]. *Asian Journal of Andrology* 21, no. 3 (May-Jun 2019): 296-99.

Marques, V., M. B. Afonso, N. Bierig, F. Duarte-Ramos, A. Santos-Laso, R. Jimenez-Aguero, E. Eizaguirre, Bujanda, L., Pareja, M. J., Luís, R., Costa, A., Machado, M. V., Alonso, C., Arretxe, E., Alustiza, J. M., Krawczyk, M., Lammert, F., Tiniakos, D. G., Flehmig, B., Helena Cortez-Pinto, Jesus M. Banales, Rui E. Castro1 Andrea Normann, Cecília M. P. Rodrigues, C. M. P. "Adiponectin, Leptin, and Igf-1 Are Useful Diagnostic and Stratification Biomarkers of Nafld." [In English]. *Frontiers in Medicine* 8 (Jun 23 2021).

Maures, T. J., J. H. Kurzer, and C. Carter-Su. "Sh2b1 (Sh2-B) and Jak2: A Multifunctional Adaptor Protein and Kinase Made for Each Other." *Trends Endocrinol Metab* 18, no. 1 (Jan-Feb 2007): 38-45.

Minokoshi, Y., C. Toda, and S. Okamoto. "Regulatory Role of Leptin in Glucose and Lipid Metabolism in Skeletal Muscle." *Indian J Endocrinol Metab* 16, no. Suppl 3 (Dec 2012): S562-8.

Mirshamsi, S., H. A. Laidlaw, K. Ning, E. Anderson, L. A. Burgess, A. Gray, C. Sutherland, and M. L. Ashford. "Leptin and Insulin Stimulation of Signalling Pathways in Arcuate Nucleus Neurones: Pi3k Dependent Actin Reorganization and Katp Channel Activation." *BMC Neurosci* 5 (Dec 6 2004): 54.

Miyamoto, L., K. Ebihara, T. Kusakabe, D. Aotani, S. Yamamoto-Kataoka, T. Sakai, M. Aizawa-Abe, Yuji Yamamoto, Junji Fujikura, Tatsuya Hayashi, Kiminori Hosoda, Kazuwa Nakao. "Leptin Activates Hepatic 5'-Amp-Activated Protein Kinase through Sympathetic Nervous System and Alpha1-Adrenergic Receptor: A Potential Mechanism for Improvement of Fatty Liver in Lipodystrophy by Leptin." *J Biol Chem* 287, no. 48 (Nov 23 2012): 40441-7.

Morris, D. L., and L. Y. Rui. "Recent Advances in Understanding Leptin Signaling and Leptin Resistance." [In English]. *American Journal of Physiology-Endocrinology and Metabolism* 297, no. 6 (Dec 2009): E1247-E59.

Nalini, D., R. Karthick, V. Shirin, G. Manohar, and R. Malathi. "Role of the Adipocyte Hormone Leptin in Cardiovascular Diseases - a Study from Chennai Based Population." [In English]. *Thrombosis Journal* 13 (2015).

Paino, F., M. La Noce, D. Di Nucci, G. F. Nicoletti, R. Salzillo, A. De Rosa, G. A. Ferraro, G. Papaccio, V. Desiderio, V. Tirino. "Human Adipose Stem Cell Differentiation Is Highly Affected by Cancer Cells Both *In Vitro* and *In Vivo*: Implication for Autologous Fat Grafting." *Cell Death Dis* 8, no. 1 (Jan 19 2017): e2568.

Peters, J. M., R. Barnes, L. Bennett, W. M. Gitomer, A. M. Bowcock, and A. Garg. "Localization of the Gene for Familial Partial Lipodystrophy (Dunnigan Variety) to Chromosome 1q21-22." *Nat Genet* 18, no. 3 (Mar 1998): 292-5.

Platek, T., A. Polus, J. Goralska, U. Razny, A. Gruca, B. Kiec-Wilk, P. Zabielski, Kapusta, M., Słowińska-Solnica, K., Solnica, B., Malczewska-Malec, M., & Dembińska-Kieć, A. "DNA Methylation Microarrays Identify Epigenetically Regulated Lipid Related Genes in Obese Patients with Hypercholesterolemia." *Mol Med* 26, no. 1 (Oct 7 2020): 93.

Rutkowska, L., D. Salachna, K. Lewandowski, A. Lewinski, and A. Gach. "Familial Partial Lipodystrophy-Literature Review and Report of a Novel Variant in Pparg Expanding the Spectrum of Disease-Causing Alterations in Fpld3." *Diagnostics (Basel)* 12, no. 5 (Apr 30 2022).

Sangiao-Alvarellos, S., L. Pena-Bello, M. Manfredi-Lozano, M. Tena-Sempere, and F. Cordido. "Perturbation of Hypothalamic Microrna Expression Patterns in Male Rats after Metabolic Distress: Impact of Obesity and Conditions of Negative Energy Balance." *Endocrinology* 155, no. 5 (May 2014): 1838-50.

Tartaglia, L. A., M. Dembski, X. Weng, N. H. Deng, J. Culpepper, R. Devos, G. J. Richards, Campfield, L. A., Clark, F. T., Deeds, J., Muir, C., Sanker, S., Moriarty, A., Moore, K. J., Smutko, J. S., Mays, G. G., Wool, E. A., Monroe, C. A., & Tepper, R. I. "Identification and Expression Cloning of a Leptin Receptor, Ob-R." [In English]. *Cell* 83, no. 7 (Dec 29 1995): 1263-71.

Trayhurn, P., N. Hoggard, J. G. Mercer, and D. V. Rayner. "Leptin: Fundamental Aspects." *Int J Obes Relat Metab Disord* 23 Suppl 1 (Feb 1999): 22-8.

Vaisse, C., J. L. Halaas, C. M. Horvath, J. E. Darnell, Jr., M. Stoffel, and J. M. Friedman. "Leptin Activation of Stat3 in the Hypothalamus of Wild-Type and Ob/Ob Mice but Not Db/Db Mice." *Nat Genet* 14, no. 1 (Sep 1996): 95-7.

Vazquez, M. J., A. Romero-Ruiz, and M. Tena-Sempere. "Roles of Leptin in Reproduction, Pregnancy and Polycystic Ovary Syndrome: Consensus Knowledge and Recent Developments." [In English]. *Metabolism-Clinical and Experimental* 64, no. 1 (Jan 2015): 79-91.

Wang, Z. M., E. G. Aguilar, J. I. Luna, C. Dunai, L. T. Khuat, C. T. Le, A. Mirsoian, Minnar, C. M., Stoffel, K. M., Sturgill, I. R., Grossenbacher, S. K., Withers, S. S., Rebhun, R. B., Hartigan-O'Connor, D. J., Méndez-Lagares, G., Tarantal, A. F., Isseroff, R. R., Griffith, T. S., Schalper, K. A., Monjazeb, A. M. "Paradoxical Effects of Obesity on T Cell Function During Tumor Progression and Pd-1 Checkpoint Blockade." [In English]. *Nature Medicine* 25, no. 1 (Jan 2019): 141-+.

Warren, M. P., F. Voussoughian, E. B. Geer, E. P. Hyle, C. L. Adberg, and R. H. Ramos. "Functional Hypothalamic Amenorrhea: Hypoleptinemia and Disordered Eating." [In English]. *Journal of Clinical Endocrinology & Metabolism* 84, no. 3 (Mar 1999): 873-77.

Wauman, J., and J. Tavernier. "Leptin Receptor Signaling: Pathways to Leptin Resistance." [In English]. *Frontiers in Bioscience-Landmark* 16 (Jun 1 2011): 2771-93.

Yang, Q., C. Yan, X. Wang, and Z. Gong. "Leptin Induces Muscle Wasting in a Zebrafish Kras-Driven Hepatocellular Carcinoma (Hcc) Model." *Dis Model Mech* 12, no. 2 (Feb 27 2019).

Zhang, J., P. P. Jin, M. Gong, Q. T. Yi, and R. J. Zhu. "Role of Leptin and the Leptin Receptor in the Pathogenesis of Varicocele-Induced Testicular Dysfunction." *Mol Med Rep* 17, no. 5 (May 2018): 7065-72.

Zhang, Y., R. Proenca, M. Maffei, M. Barone, L. Leopold, and J. M. Friedman. "Positional Cloning of the Mouse Obese Gene and Its Human Homologue." *Nature* 372, no. 6505 (Dec 1 1994): 425-32.

Biographical Sketches

Hilal Eren Gozel

Affiliation: Department of Medical Biology and Genetics, School of Medicine, Istanbul Okan University, Istanbul, Türkiye

Education: Molecular Medicine at Aziz Sancar Institute of Experimental Medicine, Istanbul University, Türkiye

Business Address: Tepeören Mahallesi Tuzla Kampüsü, Istanbul Okan University, 34959 Tuzla/İstanbul, Türkiye

Research and Professional Experience:

Istanbul Okan University, Faculty of Medicine 2021-
Istanbul Medipol University, Faculty of Medicine 2015-2021

Publications from the Last 3 Years:

1. Eren Gozel, H., Kök, K., Ozlen, F., Isler, C., & Pence, S. (2021). A novel insight into differential expression profiles of sporadic cerebral cavernous malformation patients with different symptoms. *Scientific Reports*, *11*(1), 19351.

Müge Atiş Ceylan

Affiliation: Department of Medical Biology and Genetics, School of Medicine, Istanbul Okan University, Istanbul, Türkiye

Education: PhD. in Molecular and Cellular Medicine Doctorate Program, School of Medicine, Koç University, Istanbul, Türkiye

Business Address: Tepeören Mahallesi Tuzla Kampüsü, Istanbul Okan University, 34959 Tuzla/İstanbul, Türkiye

Research and Professional Experience:

- 2023-02-20 to present | Asst. prof. dr. (Medical Biology and Genetics) Employment, İstanbul Okan University Medical School: Istanbul, TR
- 2021-09-26 to 2022-01-20 | Part-time Instructor (Health Sciences) Employment, Haliç University: Istanbul, TR
- 2019-12-16 to 2020-07-01 | Postdoctoral Researcher (Pharmacology) Employment, Centre de recherche du CHU Sainte-Justine: Montreal, QC, CA

Professional Appointments:

Honors:

Publications from the Last 3 Years:

1. Muge Atis, Uğur Akcan, Deniz Altunsu, Ecem Ayvaz, Canan Uğur Yılmaz, Deniz Sarıkaya, Arzu Temizyürek, Bülent Ahıshalı, Hélène Girouard, Mehmet Kaya. *Targeting the blood–brain barrier disruption in hypertension by ALK5/TGF-B type I receptor inhibitor SB-431542 and dynamin inhibitor dynasore.* Brain Research. Volume 1794, 2022, 148071, ISSN 0006-8993, https://doi.org/10.1016/j.brainres.2022.148071.
2. Arzu Temizyürek, Canan Uğur Yılmaz, Serkan Emik, Uğur Akcan, Müge Atış, Nurcan Orhan, Nadir Arıcan, Bulent Ahishali, Erdem Tüzün, Mutlu Küçük, Candan Gürses, Mehmet Kaya, *Blood-brain barrier targeted delivery of lacosamide-conjugated gold nanoparticles: Improving outcomes in absence seizures.* Epilepsy Research. Volume 184, 2022, 106939, ISSN 0920-1211, https://doi.org/10.1016/j.eplepsyres.2022.106939.
3. Canan Ugur Yilmaz, Serkan Emik, Nurcan Orhan, Arzu Temizyurek, Muge Atis, Ugur Akcan, Rouhollah Khodadust, Nadir Arican, Mutlu Kucuk, Candan Gurses, Bulent Ahishali, Mehmet Kaya. *Targeted delivery of lacosamide-conjugated gold nanoparticles into the brain in temporal lobe epilepsy in rats.* Life Sciences. Volume 257, 2020, 118081, ISSN 0024-3205, https://doi.org/10.1016/j.lfs.2020.118081.

Index

A

activator of transcription (STAT), 6, 7, 12, 13, 32, 33, 34, 48, 53, 54, 61, 62, 84, 86, 89, 91, 106, 107, 125, 127, 138, 142, 144
Alzheimer, 12, 13, 14, 17, 23, 27, 115
animal(s), 8, 10, 14, 23, 40, 61, 63, 64, 69, 71, 72, 81, 85, 87, 99, 101, 102, 104, 105, 106, 107, 108, 111, 112, 125, 148, 155
atherosclerosis, 41, 42, 43, 60, 67, 68, 70, 71, 73, 76

B

behavioral, vii, 1, 2, 17
behavioral and neurological disorders, 2
biochemical, vii, 21, 29, 31, 32, 39, 40, 48, 49, 51, 57, 75, 78, 101, 102, 105
biosynthesis, 4, 57

C

cancer, vii, 39, 47, 48, 49, 50, 51, 53, 54, 56, 60, 77, 122, 125, 126, 130, 131, 132, 133, 134, 135, 136, 137, 138, 139, 140, 147, 148, 150, 152, 153, 154, 156
cardiac fibrosis, 68, 75
cardiovascular, 7, 21, 36, 41, 42, 43, 50, 59, 60, 63, 65, 66, 67, 68, 69, 72, 74, 75, 77, 78, 79, 83, 109, 110, 115, 118, 121, 122, 135, 139, 141, 147, 148, 149, 153, 154, 155, 156
cardiovascular diseases, 41, 43, 60, 65, 110, 115, 118, 135, 141, 148, 149, 153

central nervous system, 6, 7, 9, 10, 19, 22, 26, 35, 113, 142, 143, 144, 153
cerebral ischemia, 11, 27
characteristic(s), 9, 76, 126, 150
cognition, 12, 24, 27, 51, 128
complication(s), 43, 82, 85, 93, 109, 110, 112, 115, 116, 117, 118, 121, 122, 148, 150, 154
condition(s), vii, 8, 14, 15, 29, 30, 31, 36, 37, 40, 41, 42, 43, 44, 45, 46, 47, 48, 49, 64, 82, 85, 86, 91, 93, 97, 109, 111, 119, 128, 129, 141, 142, 145, 146, 149, 151, 152, 157
contraction(s), 82, 90, 91, 95, 106, 107
cytokine, 6, 12, 22, 30, 33, 34, 42, 55, 62, 63, 64, 83, 84, 85, 99, 104, 106, 107, 126, 130, 135, 137, 139, 142

D

deficiency, 20, 24, 29, 37, 44, 46, 48, 50, 52, 56, 57, 64, 65, 76, 78, 79, 105, 106, 110, 112, 115, 117, 119, 121
depression, 2, 14, 16, 17, 21, 24, 65, 113, 120
diabetes, vii, 14, 18, 20, 21, 22, 24, 26, 27, 28, 31, 40, 41, 49, 51, 55, 60, 66, 74, 76, 78, 79, 83, 84, 93, 98, 101, 103, 106, 109, 110, 111, 112, 114, 115, 116, 117, 118, 119, 120, 121, 122, 129, 140, 145, 148, 150, 154, 155
diabetic complications, vii, 109, 110, 116, 119
disease(s), vii, 2, 10, 12, 14, 15, 17, 23, 25, 26, 27, 29, 30, 31, 34, 36, 38, 39, 40, 41, 42, 43, 46, 47, 48, 49, 50, 51, 53, 59, 60,

63, 65, 66, 67, 68, 74, 75, 76, 77, 78, 79, 81, 91, 92, 97, 104, 108, 110, 112, 115, 116, 120, 121, 122, 130, 132, 133, 136, 137, 139, 141, 142, 145, 146, 147, 148, 149, 150, 151, 152, 153, 154, 155, 156
disorder(s), 1, 5, 10, 14, 16, 17, 18, 20, 23, 24, 25, 26, 29, 37, 39, 42, 44, 47, 48, 49, 51, 56, 60, 64, 78, 79, 82, 85, 92, 94, 97, 110, 114, 117, 121, 125, 126, 128, 138, 139, 150, 151
dysfunctional, 95

E

eating disorders, 2, 15, 17, 77, 91
endometriosis, 85, 94, 103, 105, 108
endothelium, 6, 42, 68, 75
energy, 1, 2, 3, 4, 7, 8, 12, 17, 19, 20, 22, 24, 25, 27, 29, 30, 31, 32, 34, 35, 36, 37, 40, 41, 43, 44, 48, 49, 51, 54, 55, 56, 61, 62, 64, 66, 67, 72, 85, 86, 87, 92, 97, 109, 110, 113, 116, 118, 119, 125, 126, 127, 128, 129, 137, 138, 139, 140, 141, 142, 143, 144, 145, 147, 148, 149, 153, 157
epilepsy, 10, 23, 159

G

gestational diabetes, 82, 92, 93, 98, 101, 104, 106, 107, 108, 110, 114, 120, 121

H

health, vii, 1, 29, 30, 31, 36, 41, 42, 43, 44, 45, 46, 47, 48, 49, 53, 55, 59, 60, 66, 75, 79, 81, 91, 97, 103, 109, 110, 111, 114, 120, 129, 132, 135, 138, 139, 155, 159
hormone, 1, 3, 4, 5, 6, 11, 14, 16, 19, 21, 25, 26, 29, 30, 31, 32, 34, 35, 36, 37, 39, 40, 44, 46, 48, 49, 50, 51, 52, 53, 54, 55, 56, 59, 61, 62, 72, 75, 83, 84, 86, 87, 88, 90, 99, 101, 103, 104, 106, 107, 108, 110, 112, 117, 125, 126, 128, 129, 130, 139, 141,142, 143, 144, 145, 147, 150, 153, 156

hyperleptinemia, vii, 36, 59, 60, 65, 66, 67, 69, 70, 73, 78, 92, 114
hypertension, 21, 42, 43, 59, 60, 66, 67, 68, 69, 70, 71, 74, 75, 76, 77, 78, 85, 120, 146, 147, 148, 149, 153, 154, 159
hypoleptinemia, 64, 119, 157

I

implantation, 82, 86, 88, 90, 98, 100, 101, 150
infertility, 43, 44, 73, 82, 91, 92, 97, 99, 104, 141, 147, 149, 150, 153
inflammation, 12, 20, 21, 29, 30, 31, 33, 37, 38, 39, 40, 41, 42, 43, 45, 47, 48, 49, 51, 52, 53, 54, 56, 63, 66, 71, 72, 89, 100, 109, 110, 111, 114, 117, 123, 138, 141, 153
insulin, 4, 5, 6, 7, 8, 9, 11, 12, 18, 20, 21, 24, 25, 26, 27, 29, 31, 32, 33, 35, 36, 40, 41, 44, 45, 48, 51, 52, 60, 65, 67, 72, 74, 76, 83, 86, 88, 91, 93, 94, 106, 107, 109, 110, 111, 112, 114, 115, 116, 117, 119, 121, 127, 128, 129, 130, 133, 136, 137, 138, 139, 140, 141, 142, 143, 145, 150, 151, 152, 154, 156
insulin resistance, 4, 7, 12, 29, 35, 40, 41, 44, 48, 72, 83, 93, 94, 109, 110, 112, 114, 116, 117, 119, 121, 128, 129, 141, 150, 151, 152

L

labor, 91, 95, 97, 99, 100, 101, 102
leptin biochemical markers, 30
leptin disease, 30
leptin health, 30
leptin metabolism, 30

M

mechanism, 4, 6, 17, 61, 68, 71, 73, 77, 82, 95, 104, 114, 115, 118, 122, 142, 144, 146, 147, 156

Index

mellitus, 26, 55, 60, 93, 98, 101, 104, 106, 108, 110, 111, 112, 114, 118, 119, 120, 121, 122, 154
migraine, 10, 11, 22, 25
miscarriage, 93
molecular, 2, 17, 24, 34, 42, 50, 51, 53, 54, 55, 61, 74, 78, 79, 83, 91, 99, 100, 101, 102, 103, 104, 106, 107, 118, 121, 126, 135, 140, 141, 142, 146, 148, 153, 154, 158
molecular mechanism, 17, 102, 142
molecular pathways, 126
mood disorders, 15, 17, 21

N

neurological, vii, 1, 2, 10, 13, 14, 17
nutrition, vii, 5, 8, 18, 22, 24, 37, 47, 55, 77, 106, 119, 120, 125, 126, 128, 133, 136, 137, 138, 155

O

obesity, vii, 4, 5, 7, 10, 12, 14, 15, 16, 18, 20, 21, 22, 23, 27, 29, 30, 31, 32, 34, 36, 37, 38, 41, 42, 43, 45, 46, 47, 48, 49, 50, 51, 52, 54, 55, 57, 59, 60, 61, 63, 64, 65, 66, 67, 68, 69, 70, 72, 73, 74, 75, 76, 77, 78, 79, 83, 86, 91, 92, 95, 96, 99, 100,101, 104, 105, 106, 110, 112, 113, 114, 115, 116, 117, 119, 120, 121, 122, 125, 128, 129, 130, 131, 133, 135, 136, 138, 139, 141, 142, 145, 146, 147, 148, 151, 152, 153, 154, 155, 157
ovarian, 44, 46, 82, 88, 92, 99, 135, 137, 140, 150

P

pathological, vii, 72, 100, 106, 115, 128, 141, 142, 153
pathophysiological, 1, 69, 141
physiological, 1, 2, 6, 8, 14, 16, 22, 27, 42, 51, 54, 64, 65, 66, 81, 82, 86, 88, 97, 111, 120, 126, 128, 141, 143, 145, 147, 150

pregnancy, 21, 82, 85, 88, 90, 92, 93, 95, 97, 98, 99, 101, 106, 107, 108, 110, 114, 120, 145, 150, 157
preterm, 95, 97, 102, 103
protein, 3, 4, 8, 15, 19, 22, 30, 31, 33, 34, 40, 42, 48, 50, 52, 53, 55, 56, 61, 62, 68, 71, 77, 83, 85, 90, 91, 100, 102, 105, 107, 108, 117, 126, 127, 129, 130, 142, 152, 156
psychiatric disorders, 14
puberty, 4, 7, 17, 19, 25, 51, 81, 86, 87, 96, 97, 98, 100, 101, 105, 155

R

receptor(s), 1, 2, 3, 4, 5, 6, 7, 8, 9, 10, 11, 12, 13, 15, 20, 22, 30, 31, 33, 34, 37, 38, 45, 47, 49, 61, 71, 78, 81, 82, 83, 84, 85, 88, 89, 94, 96, 97, 98, 99, 100, 103, 104, 116, 133, 141, 142, 143, 144, 155
regulation(s), 2, 4, 7, 11, 17, 18, 19, 20, 21, 23, 24, 25, 26, 27, 28, 36, 37, 39, 41, 45, 46, 52, 53, 54, 57, 59, 61, 62, 67, 69, 74, 83, 86, 88, 101, 104, 110, 112, 116, 126, 128, 129, 132, 134, 135, 138, 139, 141, 142, 145, 146, 147, 150, 151, 152, 154, 155
relationship(s), 1, 10, 12, 17, 20, 21, 22, 24, 26, 40, 41, 42, 45, 53, 56, 60, 65, 66, 69, 72, 93, 98, 111, 122, 128, 130, 135, 143, 149
reproduction, 2, 6, 7, 8, 14, 19, 20, 29, 49, 52, 81, 82, 86, 91, 96, 98, 99, 100, 104, 105, 106, 107, 108, 128, 141, 155, 157
reproductive, vii, 3, 4, 19, 23, 26, 35, 43, 44, 48, 56, 62, 81, 82, 83, 85, 86, 91, 92, 94, 96, 97, 98, 99, 100, 101, 102, 103, 104, 106, 108, 113, 128, 137, 154, 155
resistance, vii, 10, 11, 14, 18, 19, 20, 21, 23, 26, 29, 31, 36, 37, 40, 41, 43, 44, 48, 51, 52, 55, 60, 61, 64, 65, 66, 67, 69, 70, 74, 76, 79, 83, 86, 104, 105, 111, 112, 113, 114, 116, 117, 118, 120, 122, 125, 129, 134, 145, 150, 154, 156, 157

S

schizophrenia, 2, 16, 17, 26, 42, 54
secretion, 2, 4, 5, 16, 24, 27, 36, 40, 45, 46, 55, 61, 62, 75, 78, 79, 81, 83, 86, 87, 90, 96, 100, 101, 102, 103, 104, 106, 107, 108, 112, 127, 128, 129, 136
signal transducer, 7, 33, 34, 61, 85, 127
signaling, 4, 6, 7, 10, 11, 12, 13, 17, 18, 19, 21, 22, 24, 31, 32, 33, 34, 37, 38, 39, 40, 44, 45, 47, 48, 49, 51, 52, 53, 54, 55, 56, 57, 61, 62, 63, 65, 67, 71, 72, 73, 74, 76, 77, 78, 81, 84, 85, 86, 88, 90, 92, 95, 97, 99, 102, 103, 104, 105, 106, 107, 113, 115, 121, 125, 126, 127, 128, 129, 133, 134, 135, 136, 139, 141, 142, 146, 147, 148, 151, 153, 155, 156, 157

structure(s), 2, 23, 24, 27, 30, 46, 52, 57, 61, 75, 103, 104, 108, 115, 126, 128, 142
suppressor, 33
sympathetic nervous system, vii, 2, 59, 60, 62, 69, 144
syndrome, 21, 22, 31, 43, 49, 50, 51, 65, 92, 93, 97, 98, 99, 100, 101, 107, 108, 121, 122, 131, 132, 137, 150, 151, 154, 157

T

thrombus, 71, 72
treatment(s), 8, 9, 11, 14, 18, 22, 24, 25, 29, 30, 35, 37, 40, 46, 48, 49, 52, 55, 65, 66, 68, 69, 70, 72, 87, 96, 110, 111, 113, 116, 117, 118, 125, 131, 132, 134, 135, 136, 137, 142, 151, 152, 153, 154